HOMEMADE BATHBOMBS

Project Book

Learn how to make a collection of nature inspired bath bombs, salts & lip balms

10 projects inside

INTRODUCTION

There's no better feeling than a long soak in the bath, and with these scented homemade bath bombs you'll feel like you're back at your favourite spa.

To start your bath bomb making journey, we have included everthing you will need to make two homemade lavender bath bombs in this kit. We have also included a number of recipes for other beautiful bath bomb ideas.

Bath bomb making often takes a little bit of practice to start with. With some creativity and patience, you will be making lots of wonderfully unique bath bombs for yourself and others in no time!

Perfect for beginners, these recipes will teach you the basics and inspire you to experiment with scents and colours to find your perfect bath bomb combination.

They are the ideal way to help unwind at the end of the day!

KIT CONTENTS

WHAT'S INCLUDED:

- Bath powder mixture
- Baking powder
- A round bath bomb mould
- A heart shaped bath bomb mould
- Dried lavender flowers

- (Makes 2 lavender bath bombs)

WHAT YOU'LL NEED:

- A large mixing bowl
- A teaspoon
- A wooden stirrer
- Gloves
- A dash of oil, this can be vegetable, coconut or essential oils (we'll go onto explain more about the essential oils you can use a bit later)
- Cling film
- Scales (optional)

TOP TIPS

Below you'll find some handy tips to help you along your bath bomb journey. You can refer back to these for all the projects in this book...

TIP 1: MOISTURE IS IMPORTANT

Too little moisture in the bath bomb mix and it won't hold together. Too much moisture and the bath bomb will never come out of the mould. Use a teaspoon to add a small amount of moisture (water) at a time.

TIP 2: MORE IS BETTER THAN LESS

When filling the moulds you want to make sure you have enough bath bomb mixture. You want to slightly overfill and press together firmly.

TIP 3: TAP THE MOULDS

Do not twist the mould as this may cause the bath bomb to crumble. Try lightly tapping the mould on the table a few times before gently pulling the mould apart.

TIP 4: YOUR BATH BOMB WORKSPACE

To reduce mess, work in a space that is easy to wipe down and clean. We also suggest working in a space where the bath bombs can be left to dry for 24 hours.

TIP 5: WHAT COLOURING TO USE

Make sure you use water soluble colouring, specifically made for bath bombs. Gel colouring won't spread evenly.

TIP 6: SPEED IS KEY

Once you've added any liquid to your mixture, you need to work quickly to mix everything together, this will stop it from drying out before it's formed.

TIP 7: HOMEMADE MOULDS

You can use almost any shape to create a bath bomb mould, why not try yoghurt pots, silicone ice cube trays or silicone cupcake trays – just be sure to use a material you can easily remove the bomb from.

TIP 8: WHERE TO LEAVE YOUR BOMBS

Be sure to leave your bath bombs on a flat surface and in a non-humid environment.

TIP 9: DO NOT BE AFRAID TO START AGAIN

If your mixture isn't sticking together and you can't form the shape in your mould, then put it back in your bowl and start again. If you've added too much moisture then leave it in the bowl to dry before mixing again.

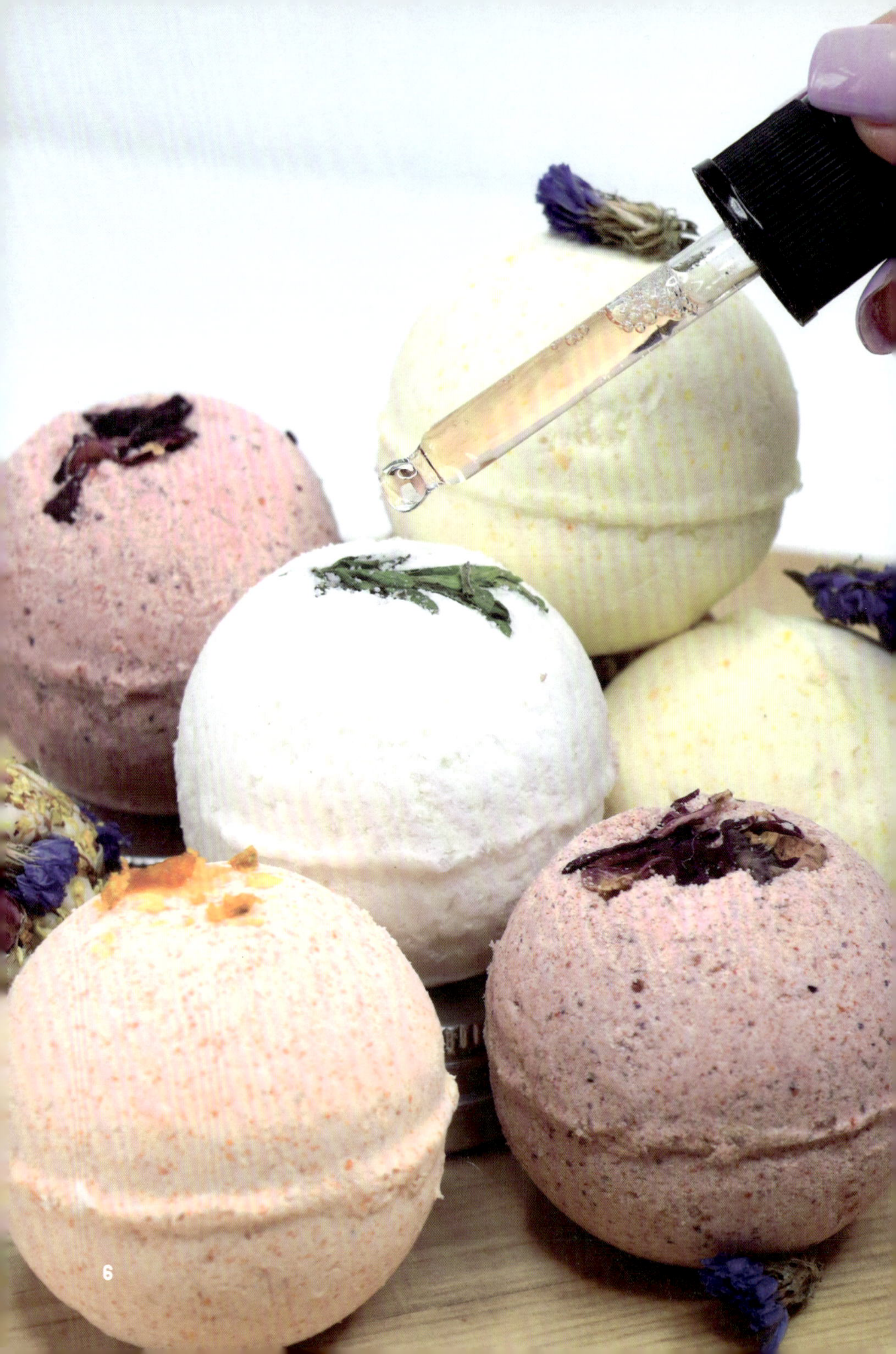

A GUIDE TO ESSENTIAL OILS:

Formed from plants, flowers and seeds, essential oils have a number of natural benefits and are the perfect addition to any bath bomb.

As well as smelling amazing and helping you to relax, bath bombs also moisturise and enrich the skin.

We recommend you test your essential oils before using them. A good way to do this is to add a few drops into a moisturiser and rub onto the back of your hand. As well as checking you like the smell, it's also a good way of testing for any allergies – remember these are natural oils and everyone reacts differently!

WARNINGS:

All the makes included in this book are designed for adults and are not suitable for children under the age of 14. Keep all ingredients and finished products out of the reach of children.

Some ingredients may irritate; always avoid contact with eyes. If ingredients come into contact with eyes or skin, wash with cold water immediately.

Wear gloves when handling the bath bombs to avoid irritation.

Do not ingest; if accidentally ingested drink water and seek medical advice.

When handling the melted oils, ensure these are cool enough before touching.

If pregnant or under the age of 10, be careful when selecting essential oils and the quantities used.

We recommend wearing old clothes or overalls and covering your work surface. Pigment in product may stain (can normally be removed with a household cleaner).

LAVENDER

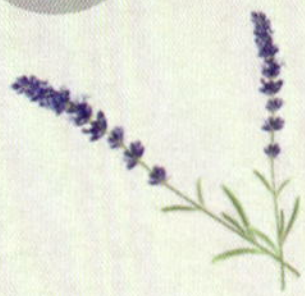

This must-have oil is a favourite for a reason. It promotes calmness, relaxes muscles and is used to aid sleep.

PEPPERMINT

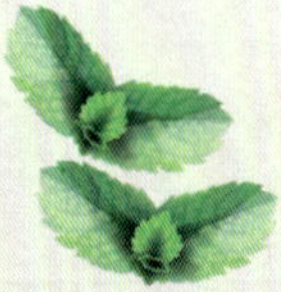

Refreshing and cooling, peppermint's powerful smell can invigorate and sharpen the senses. It is also good to soothe irritation.

TEA TREE

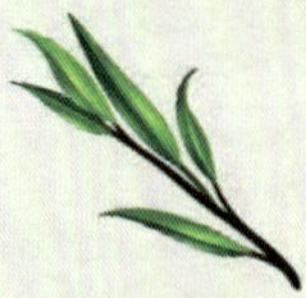

Harvested from the leaves of the tea tree plant, this popular essential oil has been used for centuries to help sooth the skin.

CHAMOMILE

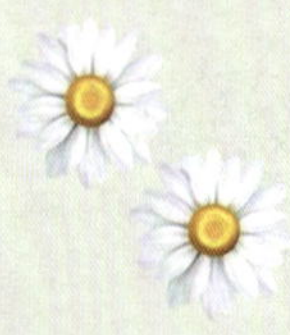

Chamomile is a herb, that comes from a daisy-like flower. Its silky texture leaves the skin feeling healthy and refreshed.

ROSEMARY

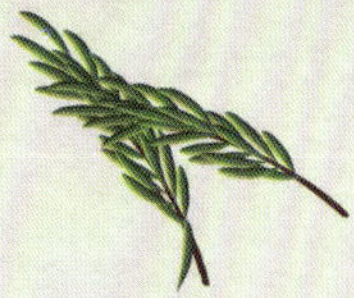

This beautifully fragrant oil is regularly used in spa products and will leave the whole house smelling distinctively fresh and clean.

CINNAMON

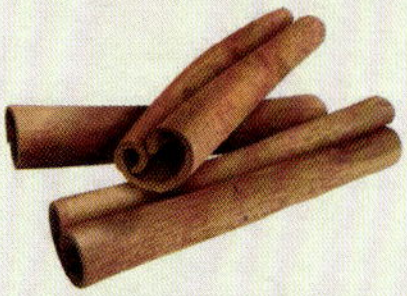

With its sweet and spicy scent, Cinnamon is used in aromatherapy for its mood enhancing and relaxing properties.

GINGER

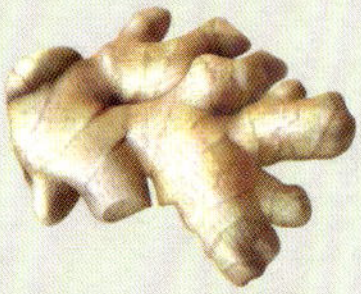

Ginger comes from a small root but packs a big punch. This zingy essential oil is said to have stimulating properties that promotes healthy skin.

LEMON

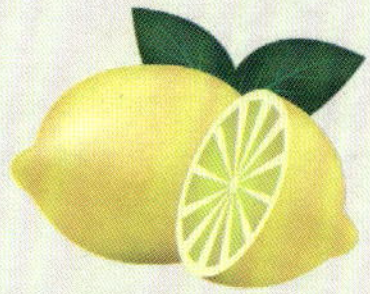

Lemon essential oil is a completely natural ingredient that is made by extracting the peel from fresh lemons. Lemon oil will leave you feeling clean, zesty and energised.

ROSE

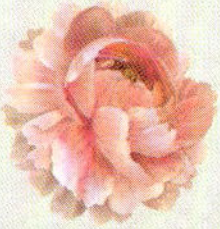

Boasting a wonderful romantic scent, rose oil is a gentle moisturiser and wonderful toner for the skin.

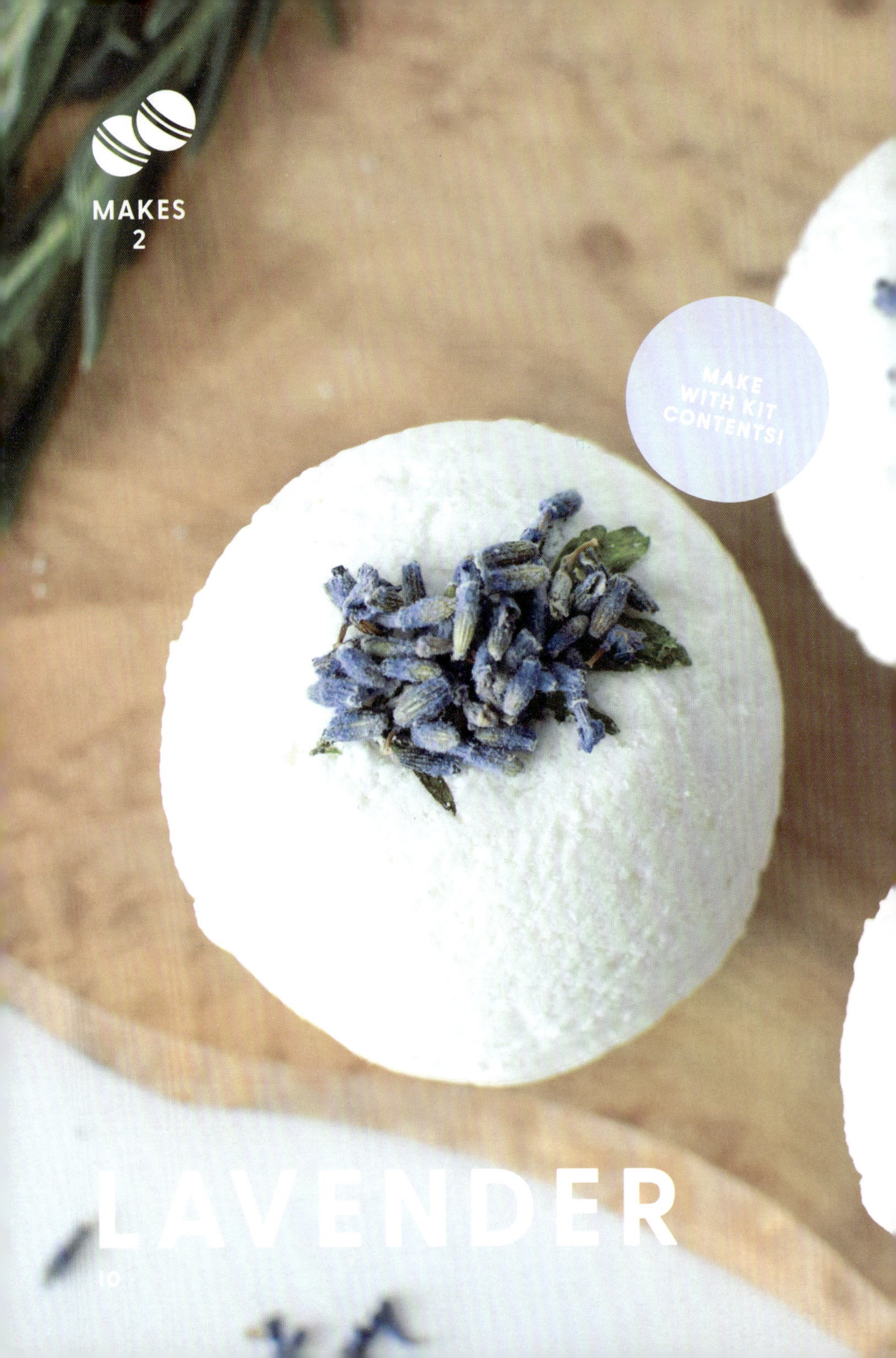

LAVENDER

LAVENDER BATH BOMB

Lavender is the perfect scent to recreate that spa-like experience, enjoy the stress relief and prepare for the ultimate night's sleep. The ingredients for this project are included in your kit and have been pre-measured for you.

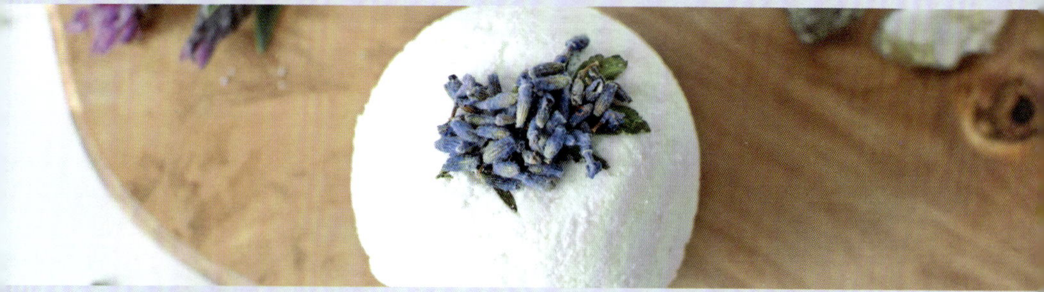

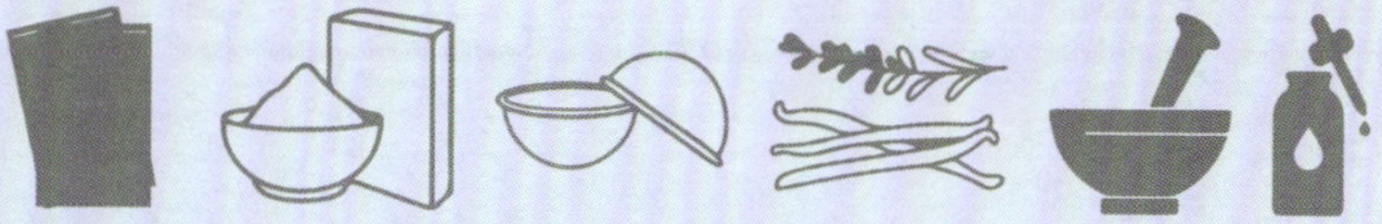

YOU WILL NEED

- A mixing bowl (similar size to a large microwavable jug)
- A teaspoon
- A wooden stirrer
- Gloves
- Water
- A dash of oil, vegetable, coconut or essential oils
- Cling film
- Scales (optional)

KIT CONTENTS

- Bath powder mixture
- Bicarbonate of soda
- Round bath bomb mould
- Dried lavender flowers

METHOD

1 First make sure you have a clean, tidy space to work in. It is best to have an old cloth ready for any spillages.

2 It's also a good idea to tear a piece of clingfilm approximately 20-30cm long, so you're ready for later in the process.

3 Put on your gloves and gently open the bath bomb mixture, be careful not to inhale the powder.

4 Pour just over half the bath bomb mixture directly into the mixing bowl.

5 Take the bicarbonate of soda and add half of this into the bowl with the bath bomb mixture.

6 Stir the contents of the bowl together until it's well mixed.

7 It's time to add the moisture to your bath bomb mixture. If you'd like the bath bomb to have a fragrance, use an essential oil of your choice. Look back at our essential oil guide at the beginning of the book to select the fragrance that's best for you. Add one teaspoon and stir well. Alternatively, for a non-scented bath bomb, use an oil like vegetable or coconut and add one teaspoon.

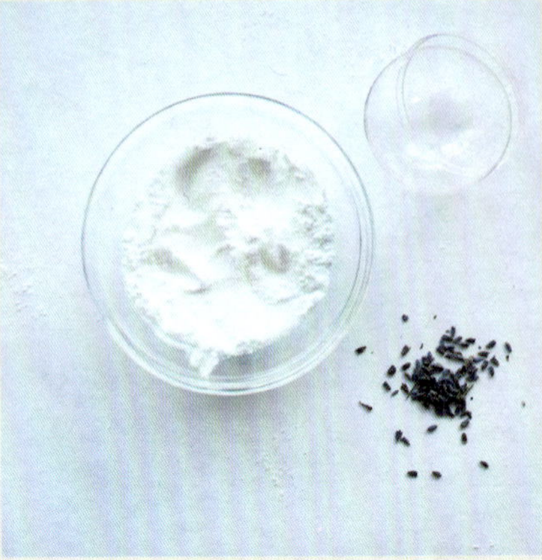

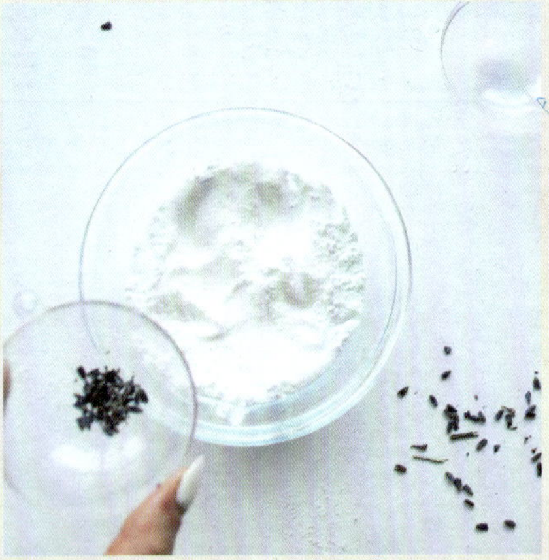

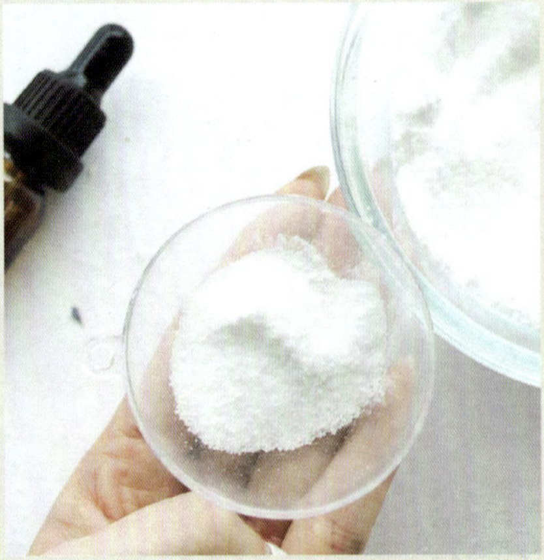

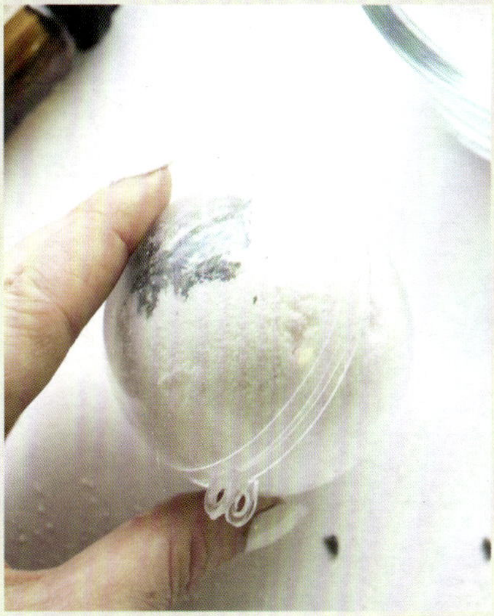

8 Sprinkle half the dried lavender into one half of your mould, try to make this a circle shape in the centre of your mould.

9 Now it's time to add water, we suggest adding half a teaspoon to the mixture first of all. Remember you are looking for a consistency similar to wet sand. Stir well and quickly once the water is added. When you add the water, the mixture will start to fizz but don't worry this is ok!

10 Now it's time to start filling the mould. Remember it's key to move quick at this point to avoid the mixture drying out.

11 Compact your moulds so the mixture fills just above the rim of the mould. We'd recommend filling just over the top of the mould but don't press it down. Leave the mixture on the top loose.

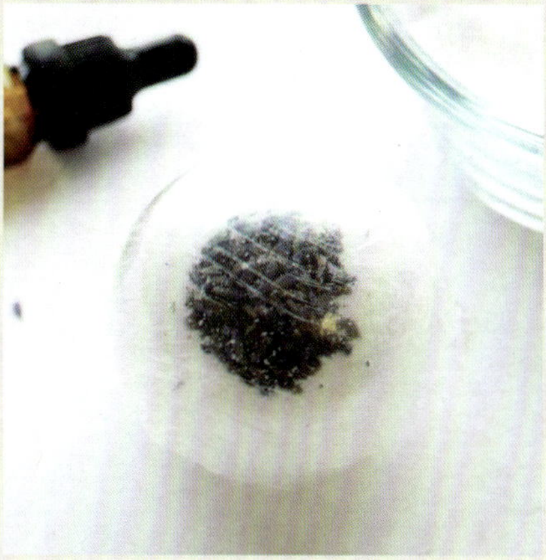

12 Place your two halves together and press the mould for 10-15 seconds. Do not twist or move the moulds once joined as this will make it harder for them to combine and could break the mixture.

13 Wrap your moulds tightly in cling film 2- 3 times. This will stop moisture getting to them whilst they set and ensure the perfect bath bomb.

14 Set aside the wrapped bath bomb and leave overnight in a non-humid area.

15 The next day, carefully remove the bath bomb from the moulds. To remove the bath bomb, do not twist the mould as this may cause the bath bomb to crumble. Try lightly tapping the mould on the table a few times before gentling pulling the mould apart. Ta da!

16 You should have enough mixture left to make this again using your heart shape mould!

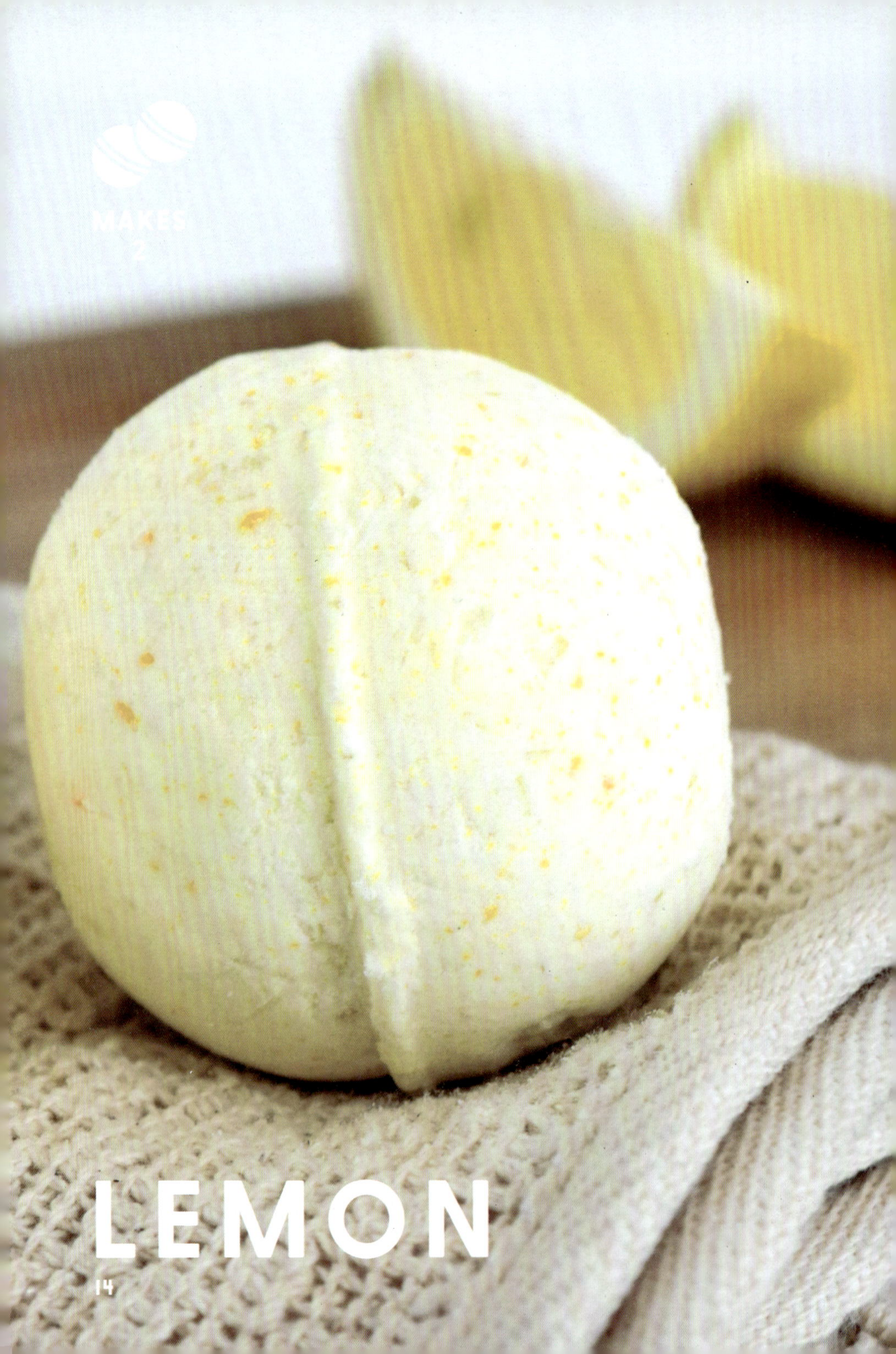

MAKES
2

LEMON

LEMON BATH BOMB

Zingy lemon bath bombs are great for detoxing and improving your skin. The lemon essential oil also reduces feelings of anxiety and helps to energise after a long, stressful day.

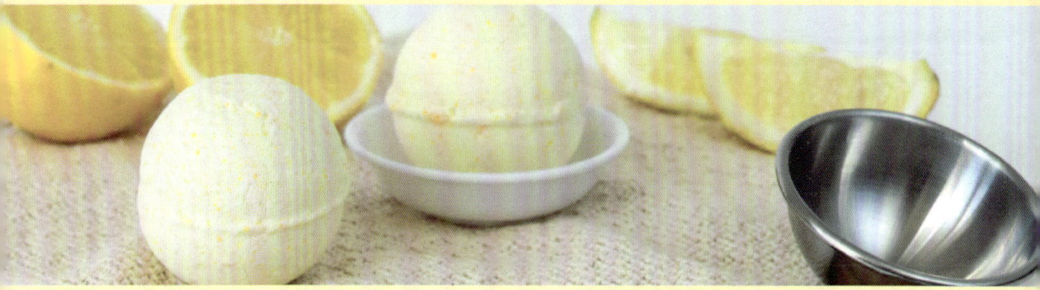

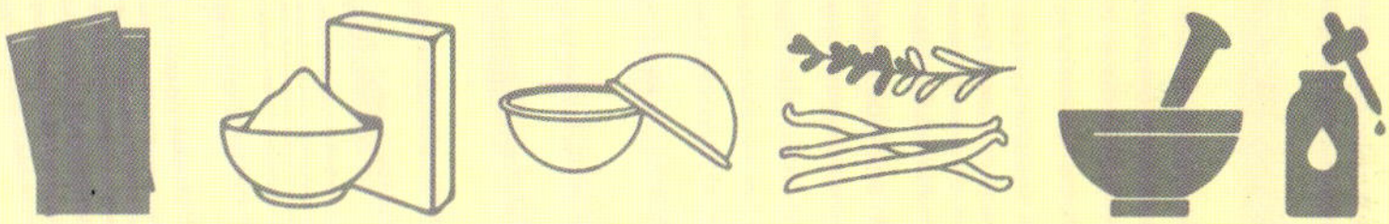

YOU WILL NEED

- A mixing bowl
- Microwave
- Microwavable mug
- Whisk
- 2 x bath bomb moulds
- Cling film

INGREDIENTS

- Bicarbonate of Soda 100g
- Cream of Tartar 25g
- Corn Starch 50g
- Epsom Salt 2 tablespoons
- Lemon Essential Oil: 6 - 8 drops
- Yellow colouring: 10 - 15 drops
- Coconut Oil: 1 – 2 tablespoons

METHOD

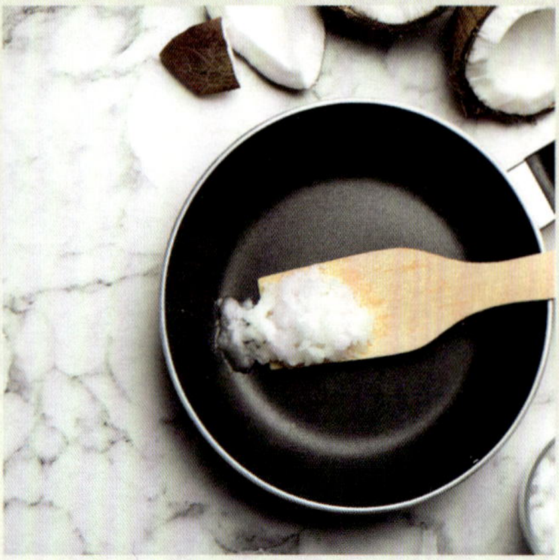

1 First make sure you have a clean, tidy space to work in. It is best to have an old cloth ready for any spillages and also have a heat resistant worktop to place the hot mug on.

2 Take your microwavable mug and add 1 – 2 tablespoons of coconut oil, 10 – 15 drops of your yellow colouring and 6 – 8 drops of your lemon essential oil.

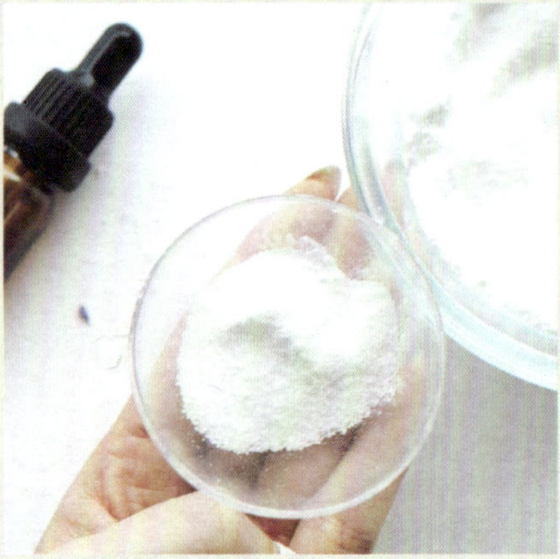

3 Microwave for 60 – 90 seconds or until the mixture is completely liquified. Make sure to only microwave 20 seconds at a time so you can check on progress. This is your oil base.

4 In your mixing bowl, add the bicarbonate of soda, cream of tartar, corn starch and Epsom salt before mixing thoroughly.

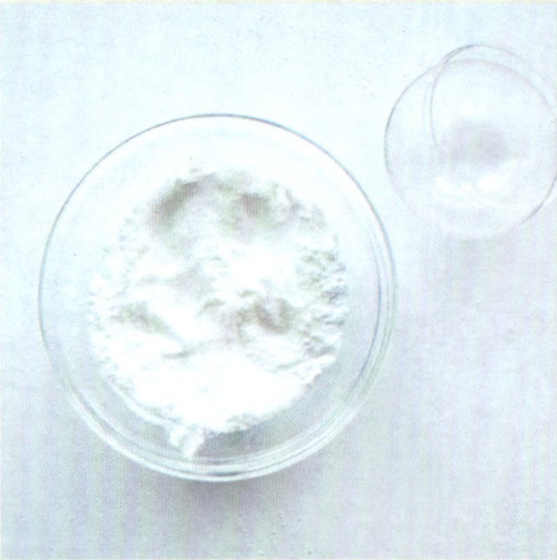

5 Pour your liquid mixture into the dry ingredients. We suggest doing this slowly whilst whisking throughout.

6 Add a teaspoon of water to your mixture and stir again.

7 Once the two mixtures are combined, give it a mix with your hands to ensure it's all mixed together (you don't want any lumps).

8 You are looking for the wet sand consistency again. If you think it is too dry then add half a teaspoon of water and mix again. If you feel it's too wet then add a couple of teaspoons of bicarbonate of soda.

9 Start to compact your bath bomb moulds and fill again just above the rim - the same as you did in your first project.

10 Place your moulds together and hold for 10 - 15 seconds. Wrap in clingfilm and leave overnight.

11 The next day, you can remove the bath bomb from the mould and enjoy your zesty lemon bath bomb!

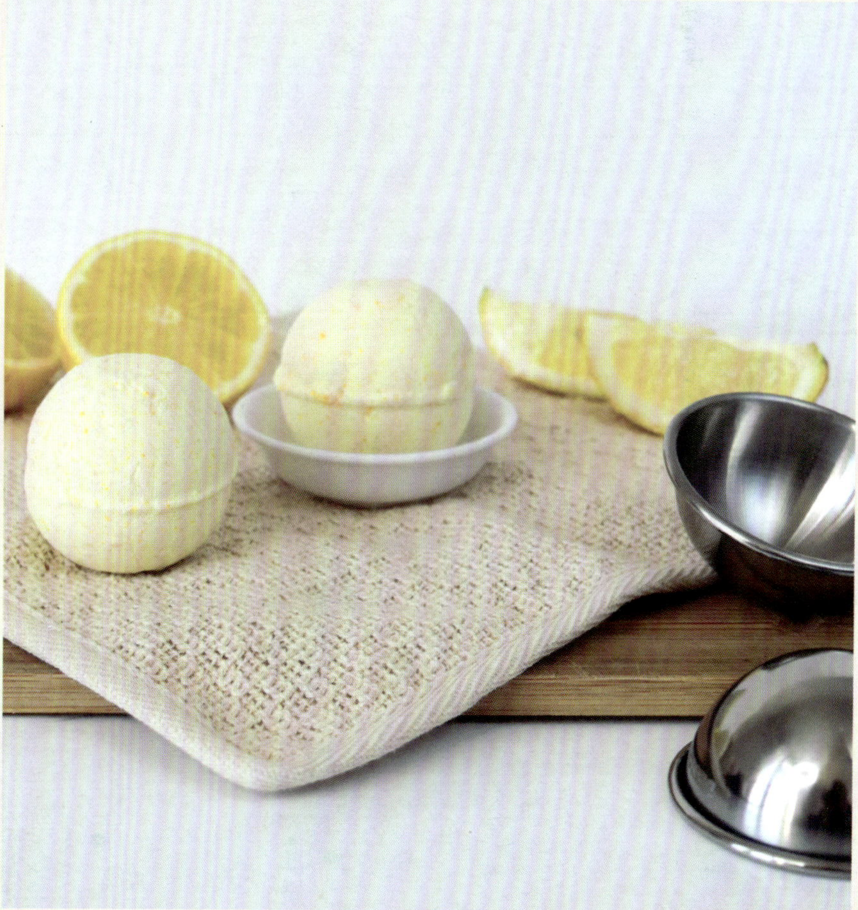

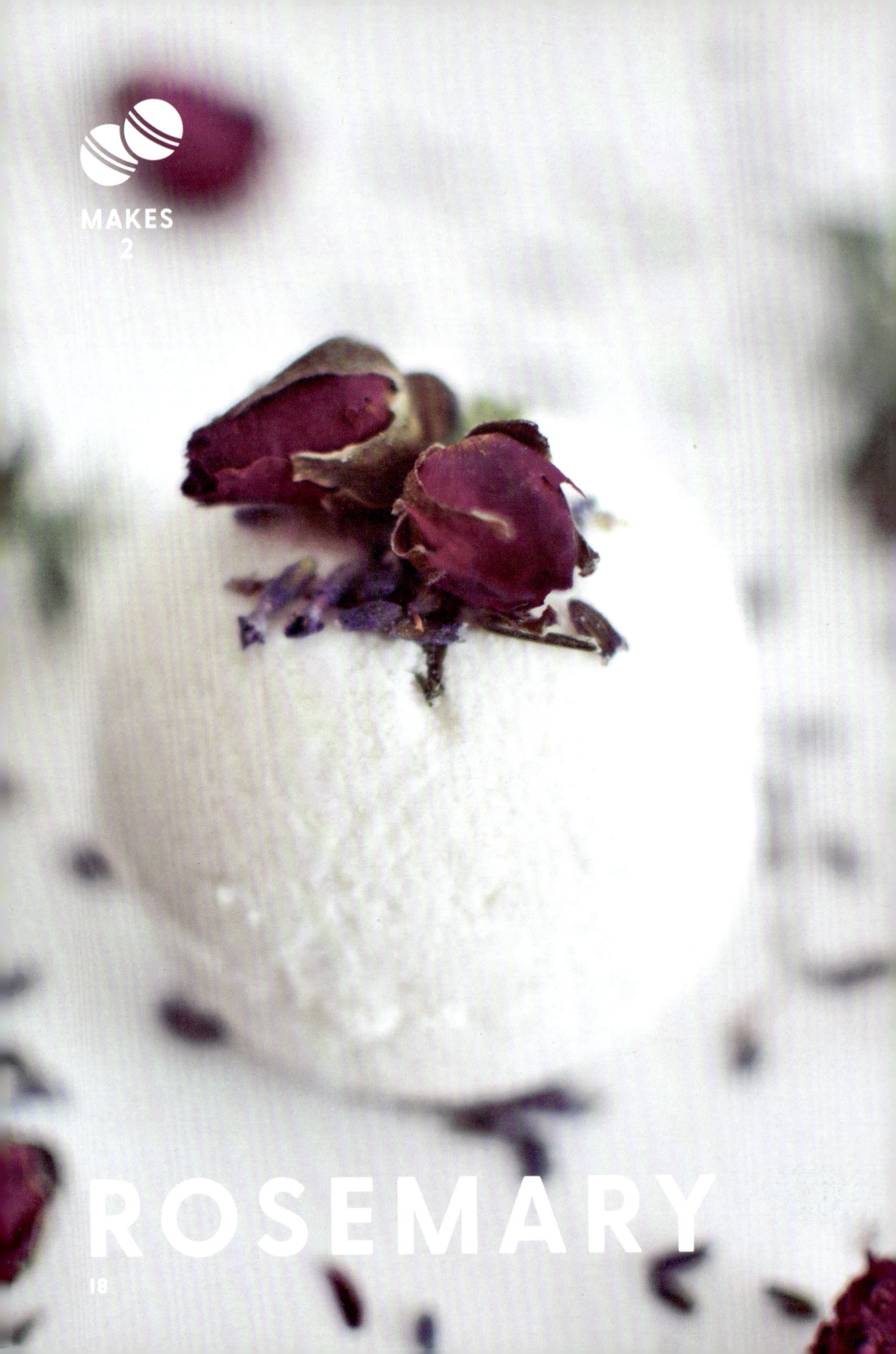

ROSEMARY

ROSEMARY BATH BOMB

A lot more than the perfect accompaniment to your Sunday roast, rosemary oil is known for supporting concentration and improving your mood which makes this the ideal prep for that busy week!

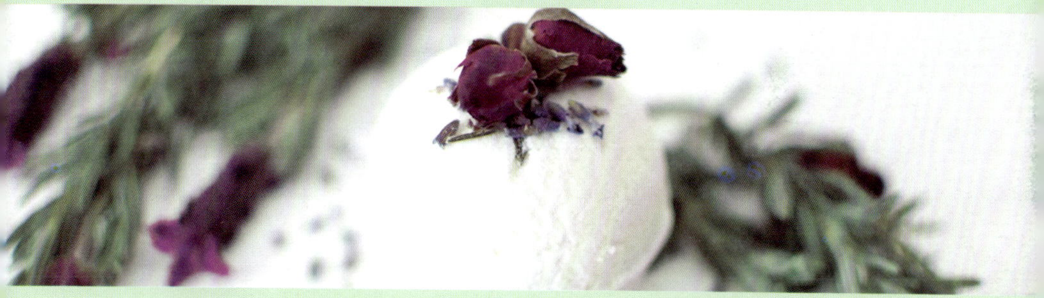

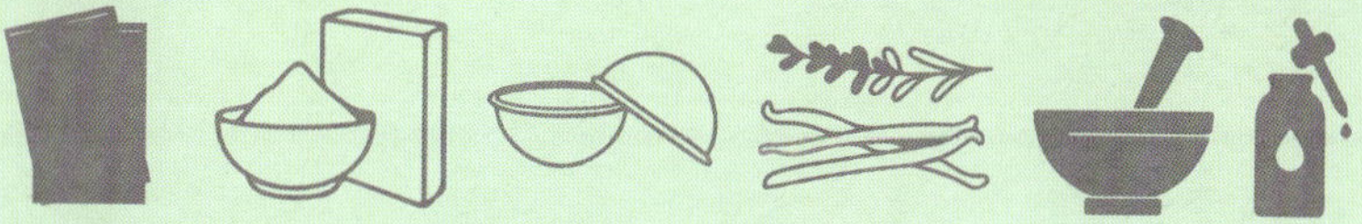

YOU WILL NEED

- A mixing bowl
- Microwave
- Microwavable Mug
- Whisk
- 2 x bath bomb moulds
- Cling film

INGREDIENTS

- Bicarbonate of Soda 100g
- Cream of Tartar 25g
- Corn Starch 50g
- Epsom Salt 2 tablespoons
- Rosemary Essential Oil: 6-8 drops
- Coconut Oil: 1 – 2 tablespoons
- Sprig of Dried Rosemary
- Dried lavender & rose petals (optional)

METHOD

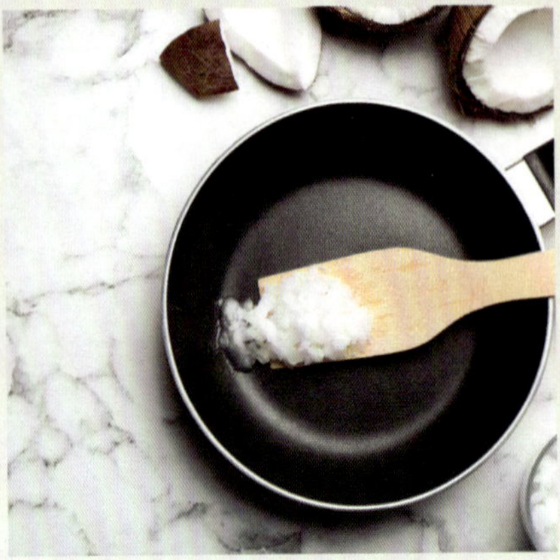

1 Always refer back to your first bath bomb and make sure you've got your work surface ready and all your equipment to hand.

2 Take your microwavable mug and add 1 – 2 tablespoons of coconut oil and 8 drops of your rosemary essential oil.

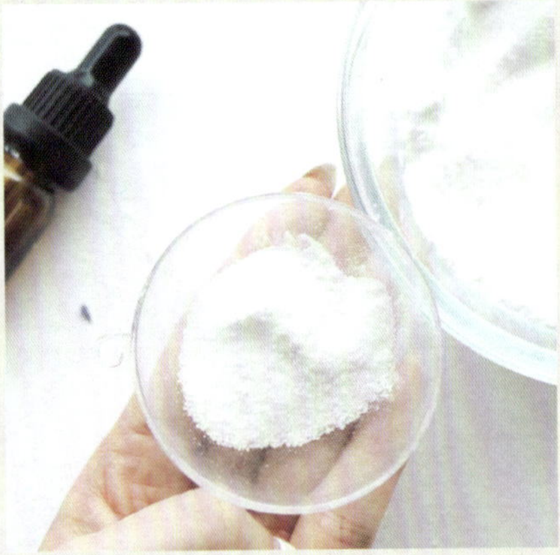

3 Microwave for 60 – 90 seconds or until the mixture is completely liquified. Make sure to only microwave 20 seconds at a time so you can check on progress. This is your oil base.

4 In your mixing bowl, add the bicarbonate of soda, cream of tartar, corn starch and Epsom salt before mixing thoroughly.

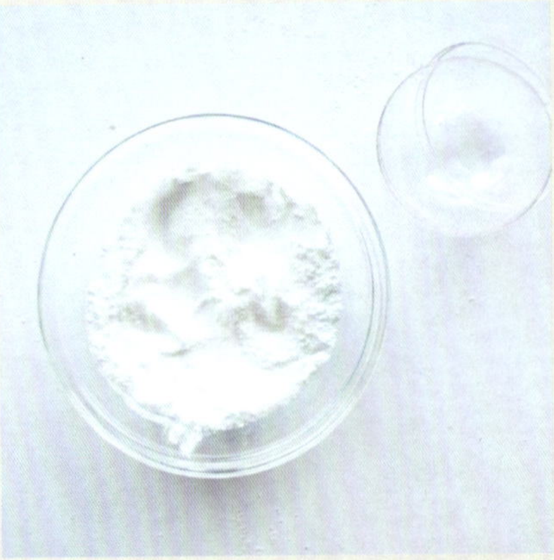

5 Pour your liquid mixture into the dry ingredients. We suggest doing this slowly whilst whisking throughout.

6 Add a teaspoon of water to your mixture and stir again.

7 Once the two mixtures are combined, give it a mix with your hands to ensure it's all mixed together (you don't want any lumps).

8 You are looking for the wet sand consistency again. If you think it is too dry then add half a teaspoon of water and mix again. If you feel it's too wet then add a couple of teaspoons of bicarbonate of soda.

9 Take your sprig of rosemary and place it in the centre of one of your bath bomb moulds.

10 Start to compact your bath bomb moulds and fill again just above the rim - the same as you did in your first project.

11 Place your moulds together and hold for 10 - 15 seconds. Wrap in clingfilm and leave overnight.

12 The next day, you can remove the bath bomb from the mould and enjoy your herby bath bomb!

13 If you'd like to add further decoration to your bath bomb, why not sprinkle it with lavender and rose petals.

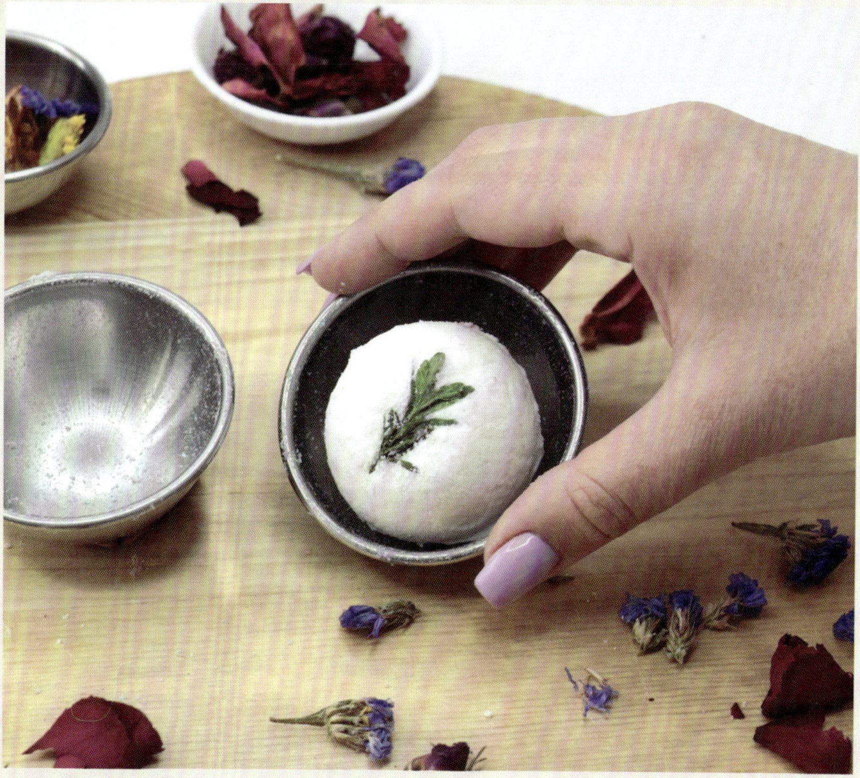

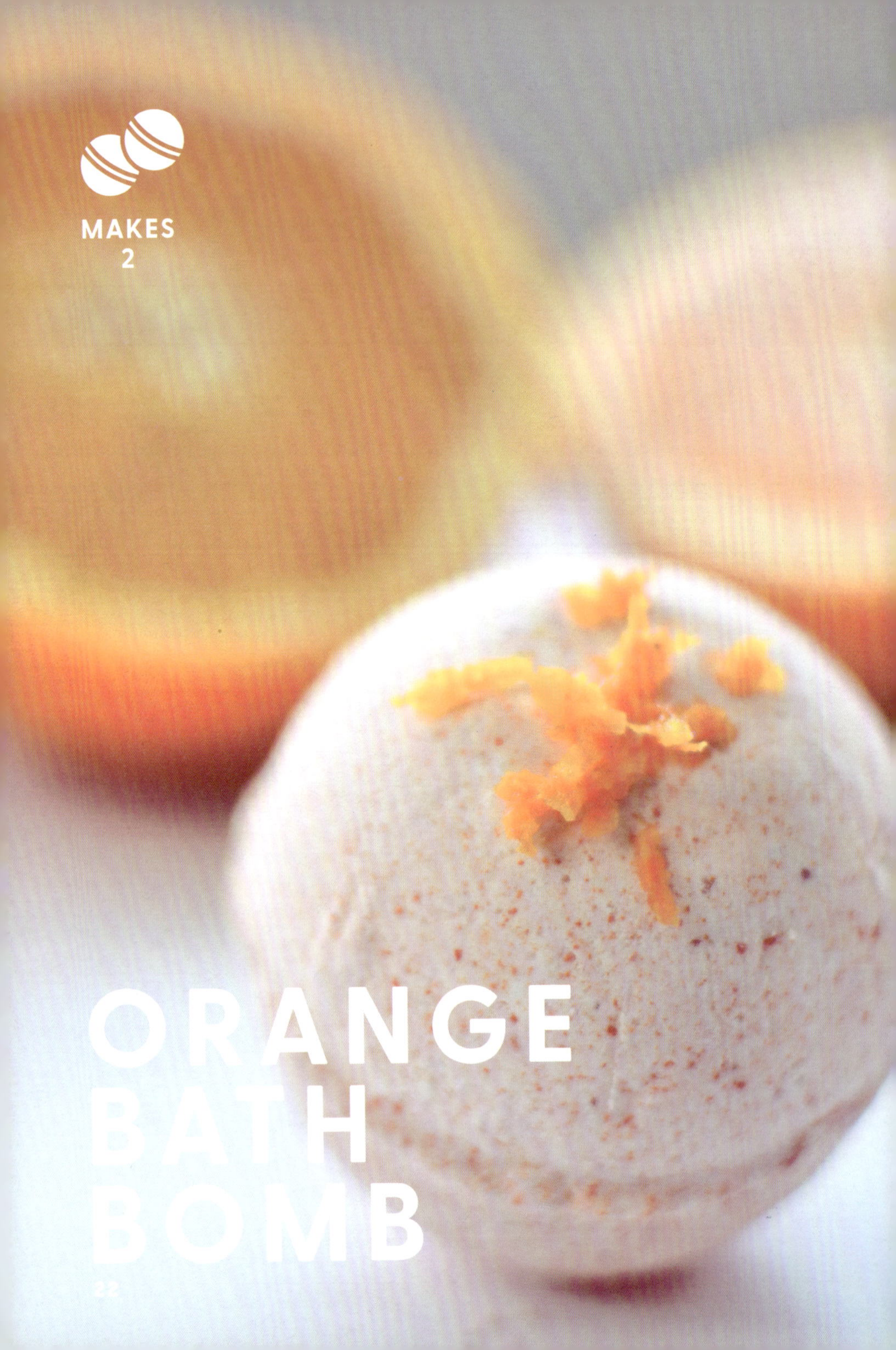

MAKES
2

ORANGE BATH BOMB

SWEET ORANGE BATH BOMB

Zesty, citrus and sweet – these bath bombs will help refresh and relieve stress after a long day. This essential oil is also known for helping treat skin conditions – an all round winner!

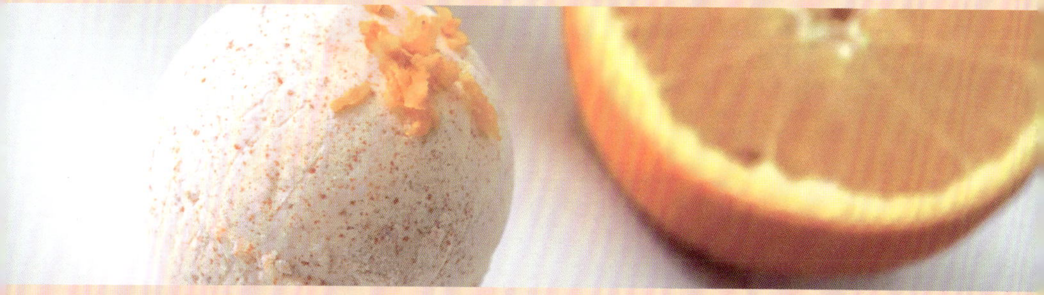

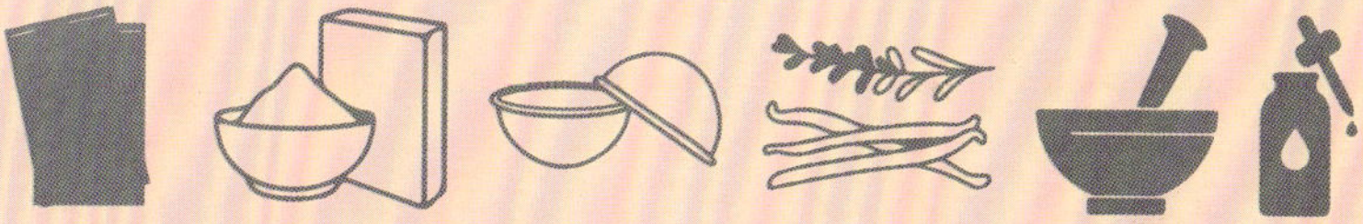

YOU WILL NEED

- A mixing bowl
- Microwave
- Microwavable Mug
- Whisk
- 2 x Bath Bomb moulds
- Clingfilm

INGREDIENTS

- Bicarbonate of Soda 100g
- Cream of Tartar 25g
- Corn Starch 50g
- Epsom Salt 2 tablespoons
- Sweet Orange Essential Oil: 6 - 8 drops
- Orange colouring: 10 - 15 drops
- Coconut Oil: 1 – 2 tablespoons

METHOD

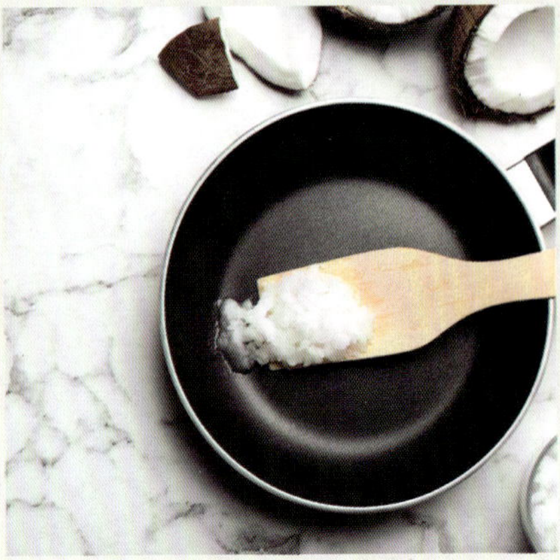

1 Always refer back to your first bath bomb and make sure you've got your work surface ready and all your equipment to hand.

2 Take your microwavable mug and add 1 – 2 tablespoons of coconut oil, 10 – 15 drops of your orange colouring and 6 – 8 drops of your sweet orange essential oil.

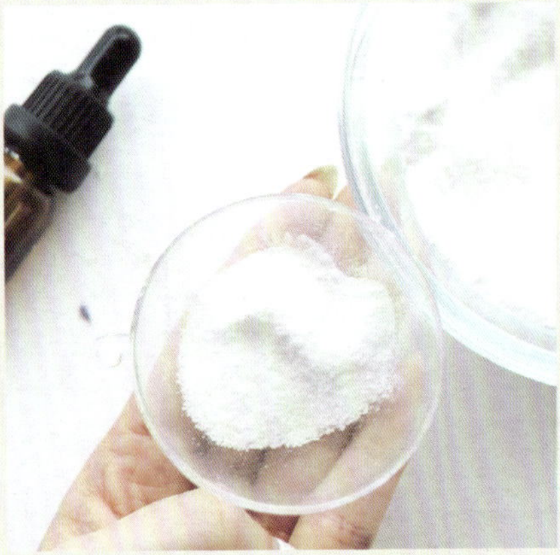

3 Microwave for 60 – 90 seconds or until the mixture is completely liquified. Make sure to only microwave 20 seconds at a time so you can check on progress. This is your oil base.

4 In your mixing bowl, add the bicarbonate of soda, cream of tartar, corn starch and Epsom salt before mixing thoroughly.

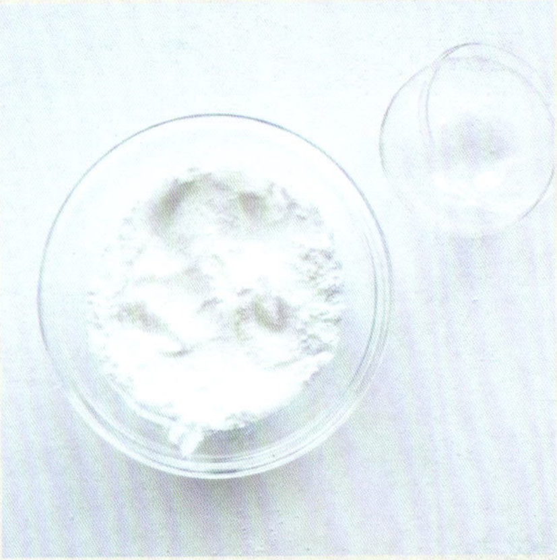

5 Pour your liquid mixture into the dry ingredients. We suggest doing this slowly whilst whisking throughout.

6 Add a teaspoon of water to your mixture and stir again.

7 Once the two mixtures are combined, give it a mix with your hands to ensure it's all mixed together (you don't want any lumps).

8 You are looking for the wet sand consistency again. If you think it is too dry then add half a teaspoon of water and mix again. If you feel it's too wet then add a couple of teaspoons of bicarbonate of soda.

9 Start to compact your bath bomb moulds and fill again just above the rim - the same as you did in your first project.

10 Place your moulds together and hold for 10 - 15 seconds. Wrap in clingfilm and leave overnight.

11 The next day, you can remove the bath bomb from the mould and enjoy your refreshing citrus bath bomb!

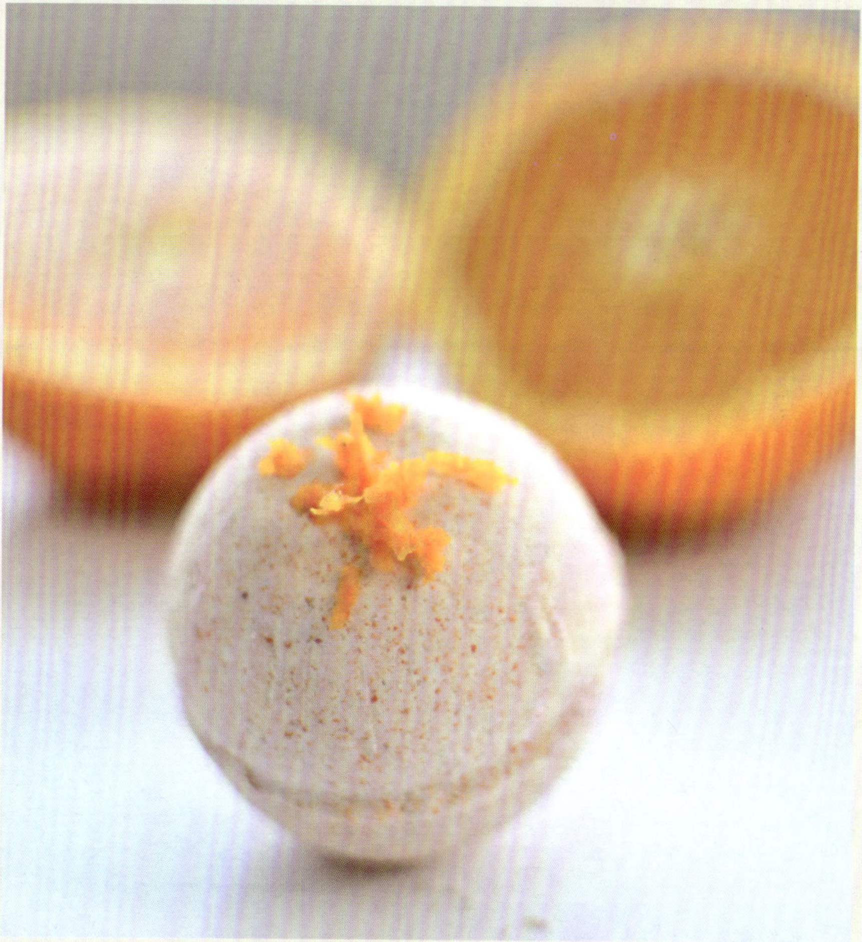

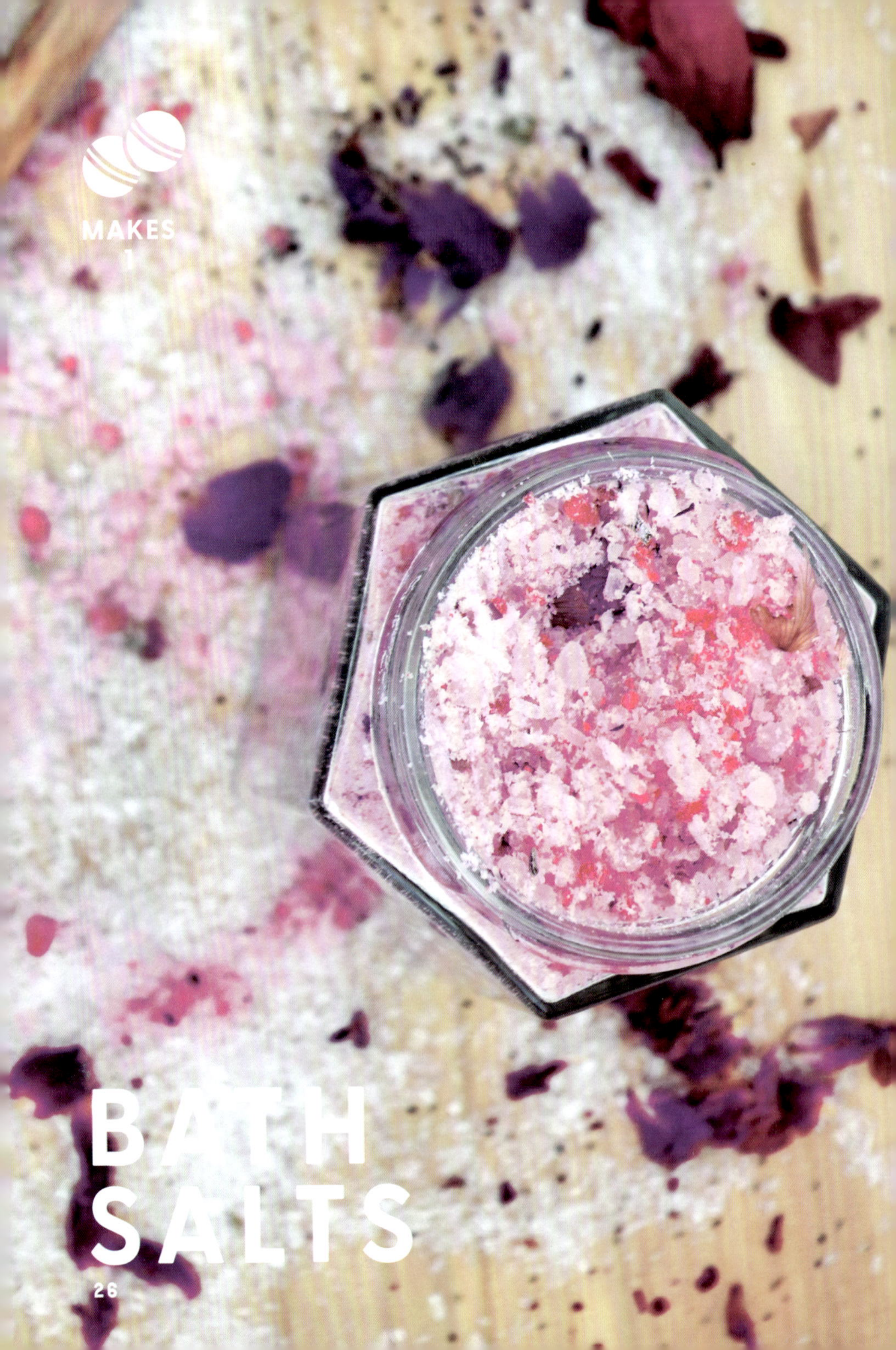

MAKES
1

BATH SALTS

BATH SALTS

A nice Epsom salt soak is more than just your average bath. The salts help promote relaxation, reduce inflammation and joint pain. This really simple recipe will give you weeks of joy.

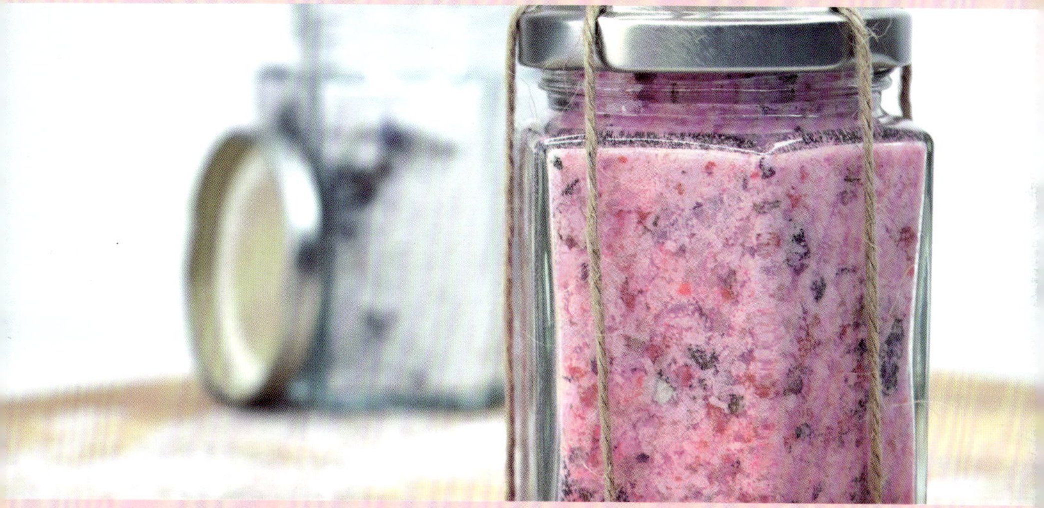

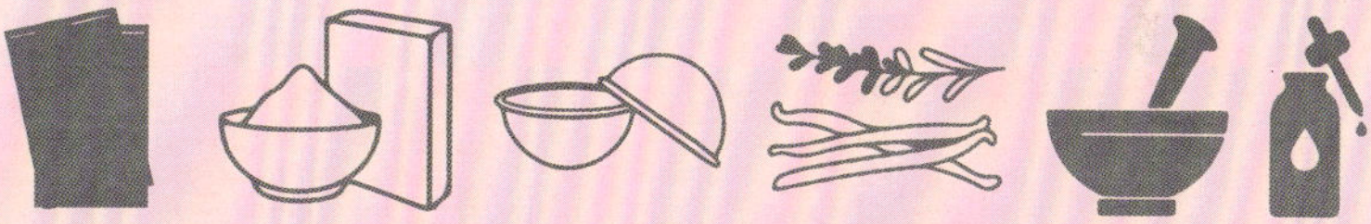

YOU WILL NEED

- 2 x mixing bowls
- Container / jar

INGREDIENTS

- Rock Salt 70g
- Epsom Salt 70g
- Bicarbonate of Soda 30g
- Essential Oil: 8 - 12 drops
- Dried Flowers (handful)
- Colouring: 3-4 drops (optional)

METHOD

1 Prepare your work surface and equipment in the same way you did on the bath bomb projects.

2 In your large mixing bowl combine your rock salt, Epsom salt, bicarbonate of soda & dried flowers, whisk until fully combined.

3 Add in your essential oil and whisk again. We recommend around 8–12 drops depending on the scent you have chosen.

4 For natural and colour free salts, just spoon the mixture into a container or jar and cover.

OR

For the coloured salts, separate your mixture equally into two separate bowls.

5 Add your colouring to one of the bowls. Start with 3–4 drops and mix, add more until you reach your desired colour.

6 Start to spoon one colour into your jar/container until you have a layer. Then take another spoon and add in your other colour. Repeat this process until the jar is full and you have the effect you are looking for.

7 Store in a jar with a lid - add some twine or ribbon to make it the perfect gift!

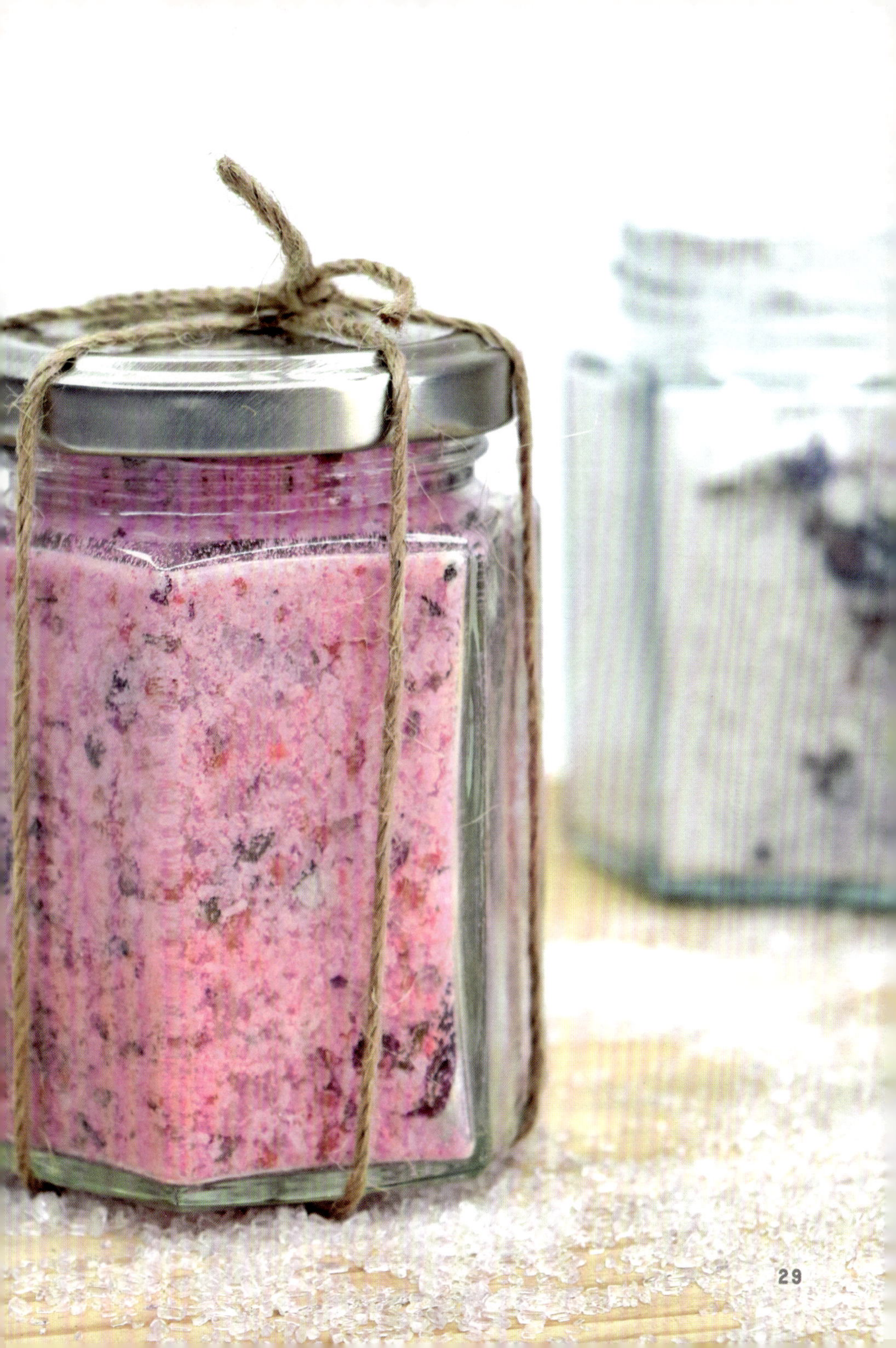

MAKES
2

PEPPERMINT

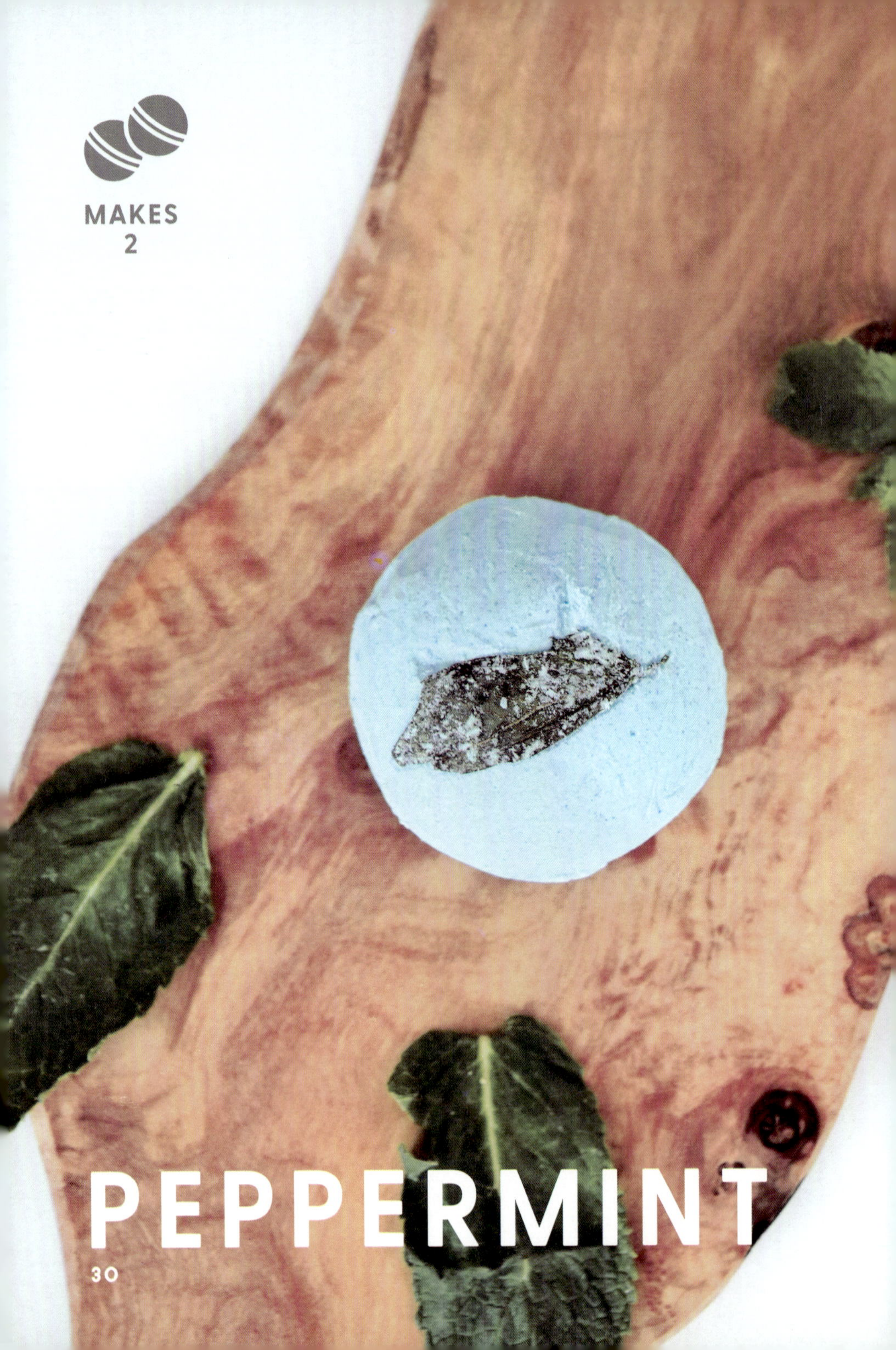

PEPPERMINT BATH BOMB

Known to help relieve headaches and stress. Peppermint creates the perfect fresh scent to help you unwind. Guaranteed to pick you up after a long day.

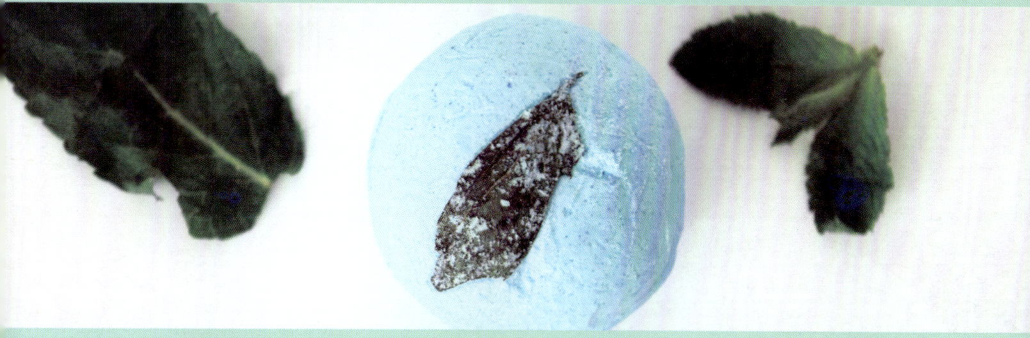

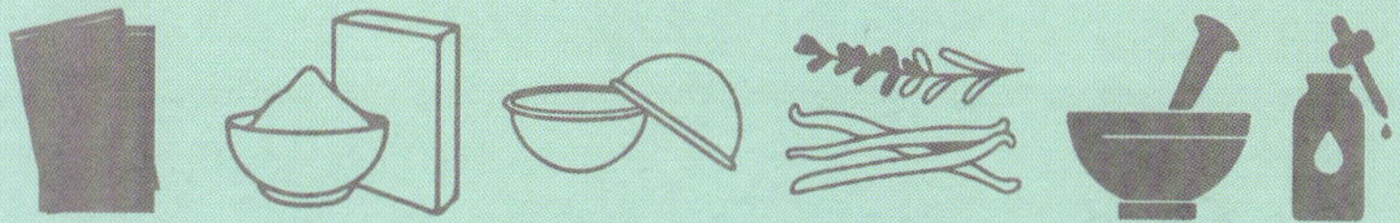

YOU WILL NEED

- A mixing bowl
- Microwave
- Microwavable Mug
- Whisk
- 2 x Bath Bomb moulds
- Clingfilm

INGREDIENTS

- Bicarbonate of Soda 100g
- Cream of Tartar 25g
- Corn Starch 50g
- Epsom Salt 2 tablespoons
- Peppermint Essential Oil: 6-8 drops
- Blue colouring: 10-15 drops
- Coconut Oil: 1 – 2 tablespoons
- Peppermint leaf

METHOD

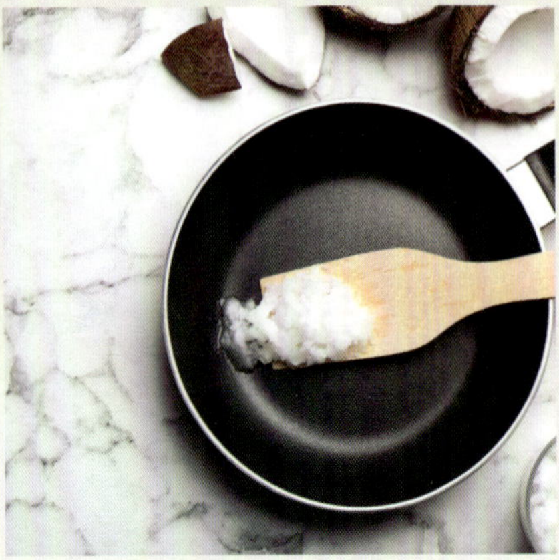

1 Always refer back to your first bath bomb and make sure you've got your work surface ready and all your equipment to hand.

2 Take your microwavable mug and add 1 – 2 tablespoons of coconut oil, 10 – 15 drops of your blue colouring and 6 – 8 drops of your peppermint essential oil.

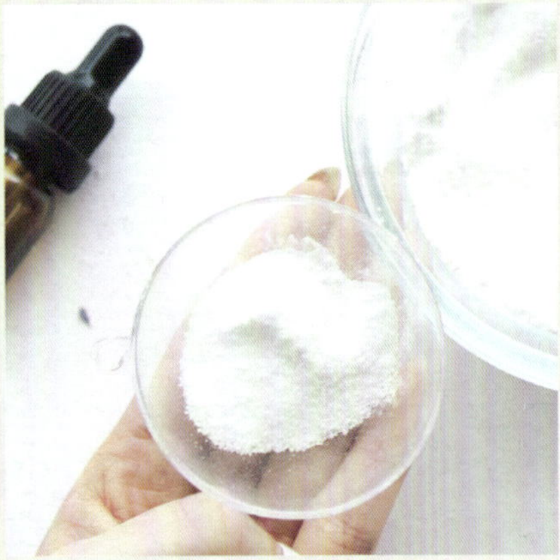

3 Microwave for 60 – 90 seconds or until the mixture is completely liquified. Make sure to only microwave 20 seconds at a time so you can check on progress. This is your oil base.

4 In your mixing bowl, add the bicarbonate of soda, cream of tartar, corn starch and Epsom salt before mixing thoroughly.

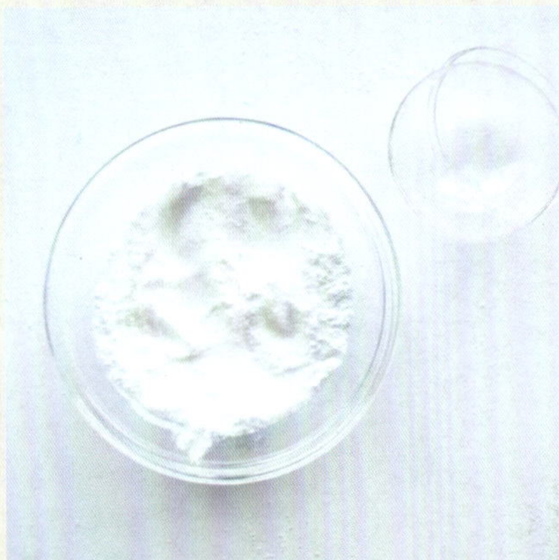

5 Pour your liquid mixture into the dry ingredients. We suggest doing this slowly whilst whisking throughout.

6 Add a teaspoon of water to your mixture and stir again.

7 Once the two mixtures are combined, give it a mix with your hands to ensure it's all mixed together (you don't want any lumps).

8 You are looking for the wet sand consistency again. If you think it is too dry then add half a teaspoon of water and mix again. If you feel it's too wet then add a couple of teaspoons of bicarbonate of soda.

9 Take your peppermint leaf and place it in the centre of your mould halves.

10 Start to compact your bath bomb moulds and fill again just above the rim - the same as you did in your first project.

11 Place your moulds together and hold for 10 - 15 seconds. Wrap in clingfilm and leave overnight.

12 The next day, you can remove the bath bomb from the mould and enjoy your uplifting minty bath bomb!

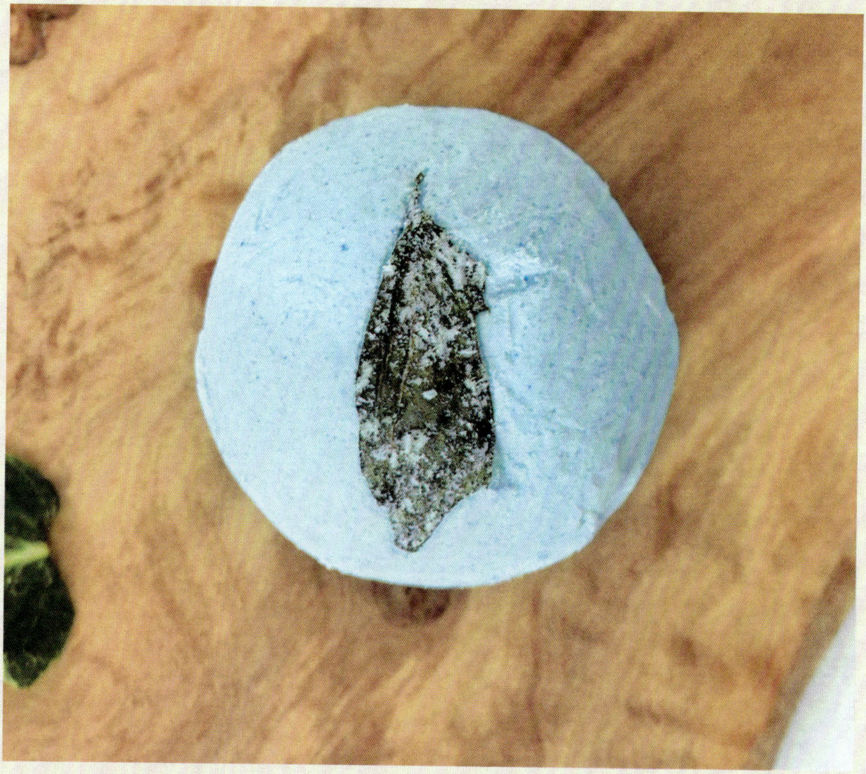

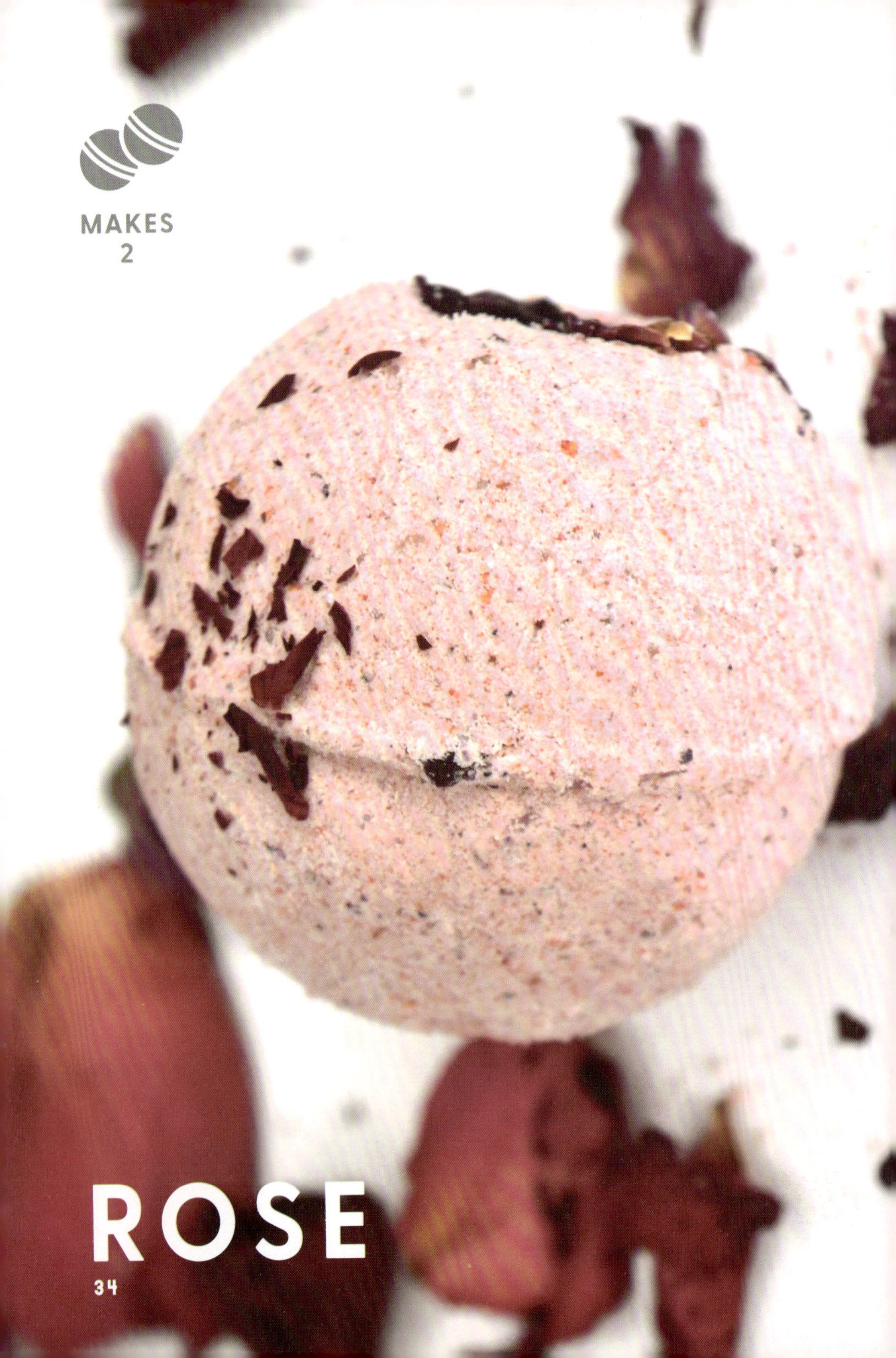

MAKES
2

ROSE

ROSE BATH BOMB

Made with sweet rose, these floral bath bombs would pair perfectly with a candle lit bath to unwind after a long day.

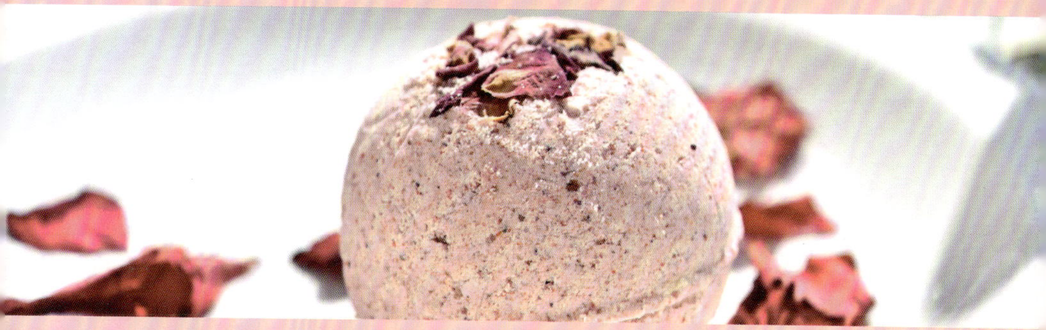

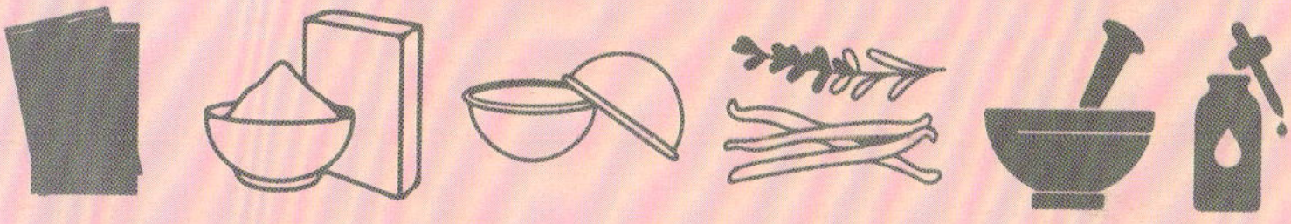

YOU WILL NEED

- A mixing bowl
- Microwave
- Microwavable Mug
- Whisk
- 2 x Bath Bomb moulds
- Clingfilm

INGREDIENTS

- Bicarbonate of Soda 100g
- Cream of Tartar 25g
- Corn Starch 50g
- Epsom Salt 2 tablespoons
- Rose Essential Oil: 6 - 8 drops
- Red food colouring: 10 - 15 drops
- Coconut Oil: 1 - 2 tablespoons
- Dried rose petals (handful)

METHOD

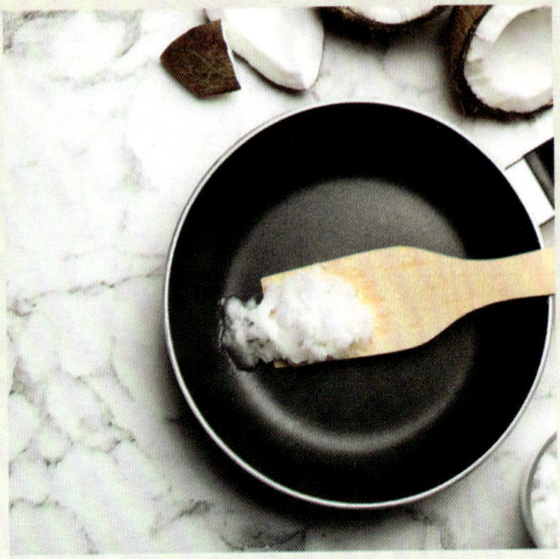

1 Always refer back to your first bath bomb and make sure you've got your work surface ready and all your equipment to hand.

2 Take your microwavable mug and add 1 – 2 tablespoons of coconut oil, 10 – 15 drops of your red colouring and 6 – 8 drops of your rose essential oil.

3 Microwave for 60 – 90 seconds or until the mixture is completely liquified. Make sure to only microwave 20 seconds at a time so you can check on progress. This is your oil base.

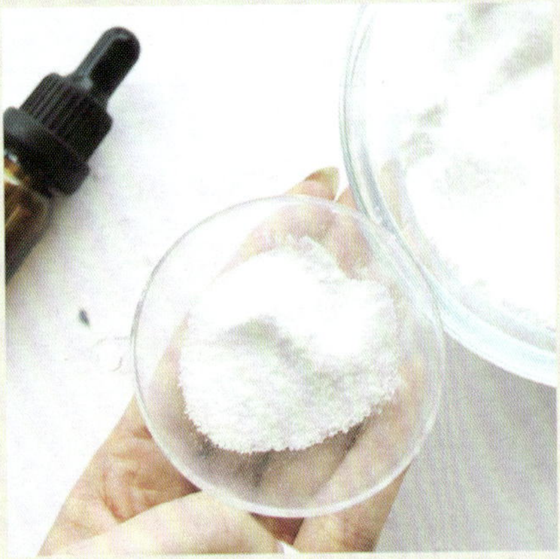

4 In your mixing bowl, add the bicarbonate of soda, cream of tartar, corn starch and Epsom salt before mixing thoroughly.

5 Pour your liquid mixture into the dry ingredients. We suggest doing this slowly whilst whisking throughout.

6 Add a teaspoon of water to your mixture and stir again.

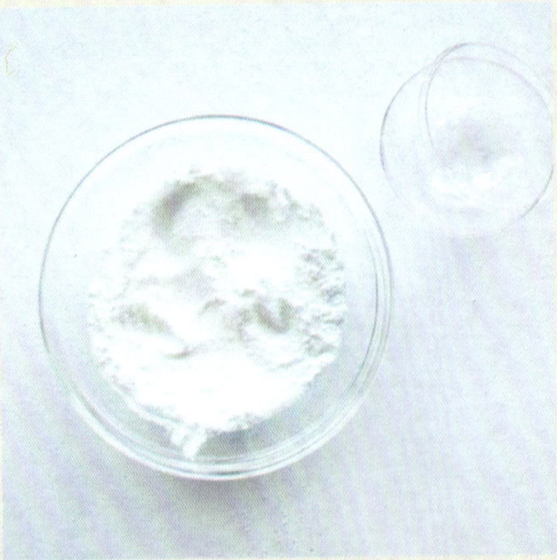

7 Once the two mixtures are combined, give it a mix with your hands to ensure it's all mixed together (you don't want any lumps).

8 You are looking for the wet sand consistency again. If you think it is too dry then add half a teaspoon of water and mix again. If you feel it's too wet then add a couple of teaspoons of bicarbonate of soda.

9 Take a small handful of rose petals and place them in the centre of one of your bath bomb moulds. Make sure there's still plenty of room for bath bomb mixture.

10 Start to compact your bath bomb moulds and fill again just above the rim - the same as you did in your first project.

11 Place your moulds together and hold for 10 - 15 seconds. Wrap in clingfilm and leave overnight.

12 The next day, you can remove the bath bomb from the mould and enjoy your beautifully floral bath bomb!

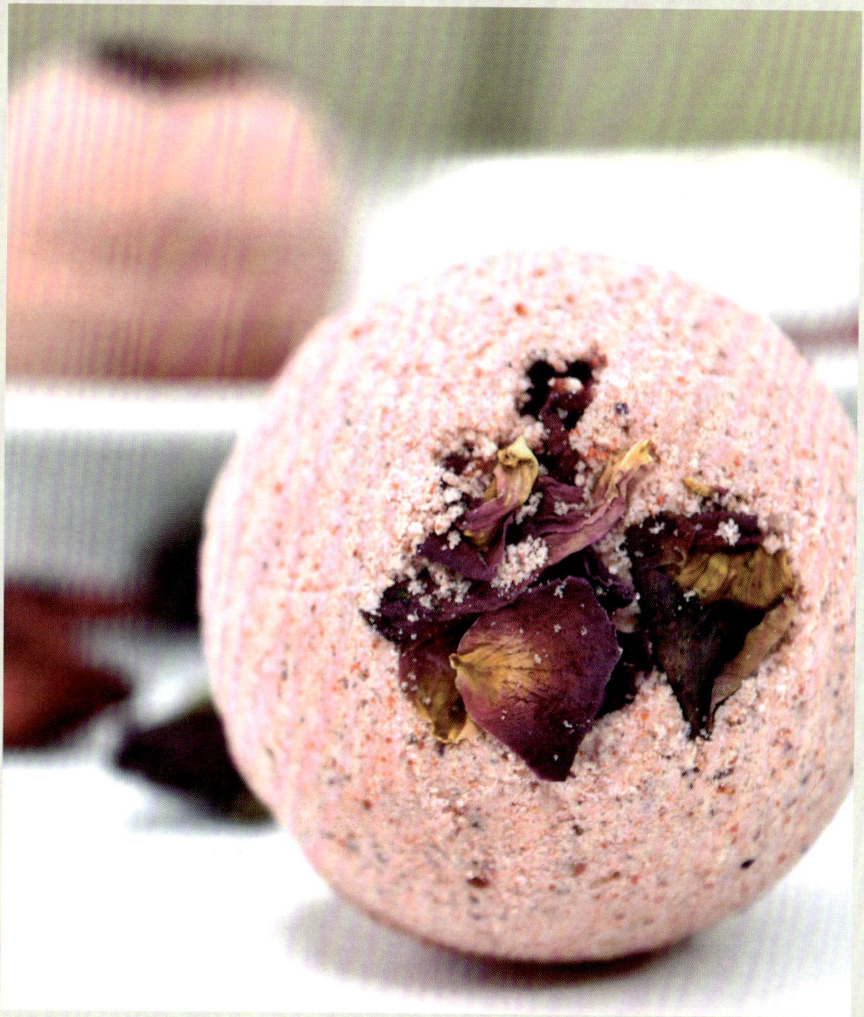

MAKES
2

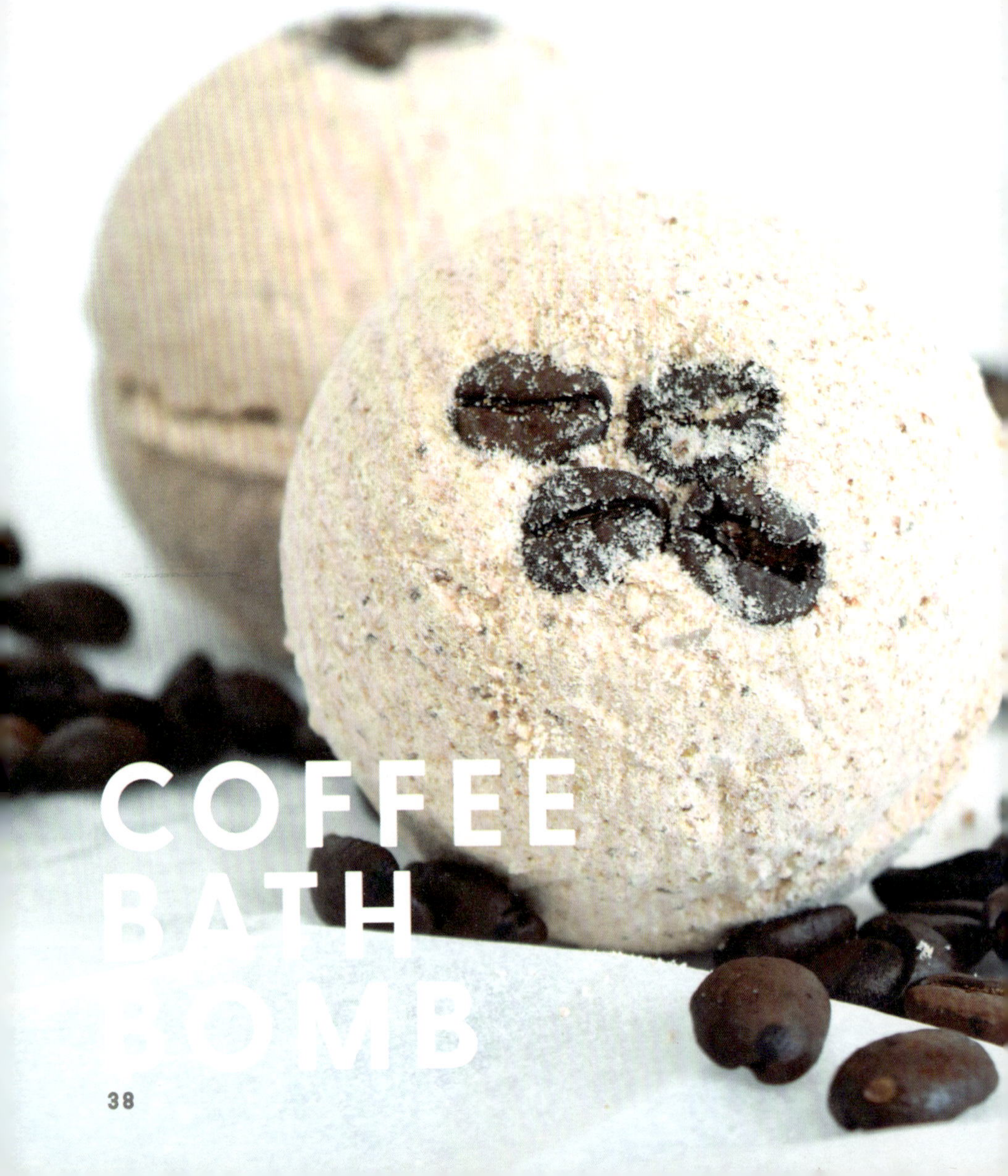

COFFEE BATH BOMB

COFFEE BATH BOMB

Just like your morning coffee, these bath bombs will be sure to perk you up. The caffeine in coffee also has a number of benefits for your skin, including reducing inflammation and increasing skin smoothness and brightness.

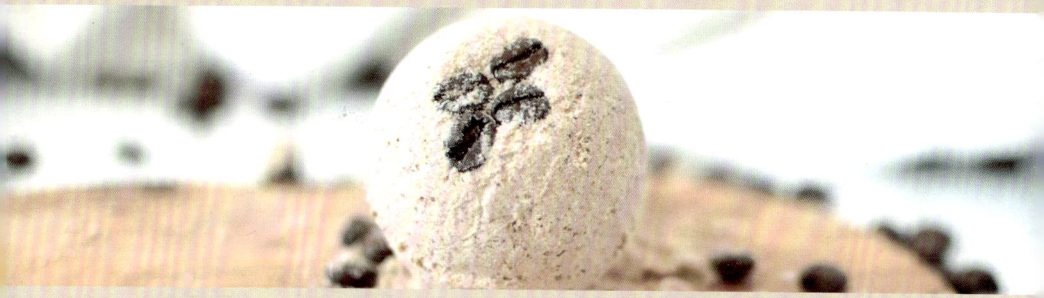

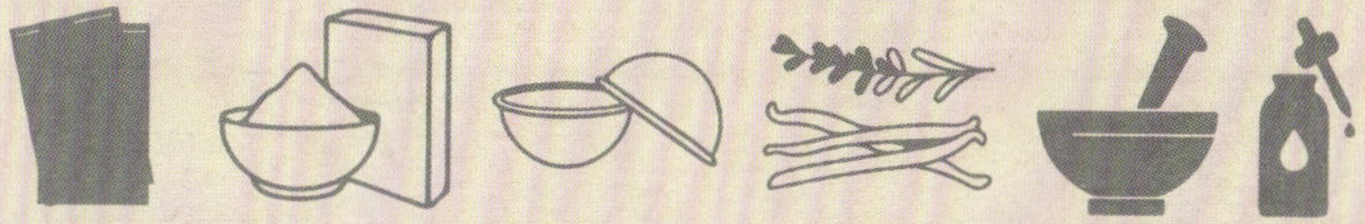

YOU WILL NEED

- A mixing bowl
- Microwave
- Microwavable Mug
- Whisk
- 2 x Bath Bomb moulds
- Clingfilm

INGREDIENTS

- Bicarbonate of Soda 100g
- Cream of Tartar 25g
- Corn Starch 50g
- Epsom Salt 2 tablespoons
- Ground (instant) coffee 1 tablespoon
- Coffee beans (handful)
- Coconut Oil: 1 – 2 tablespoons

METHOD

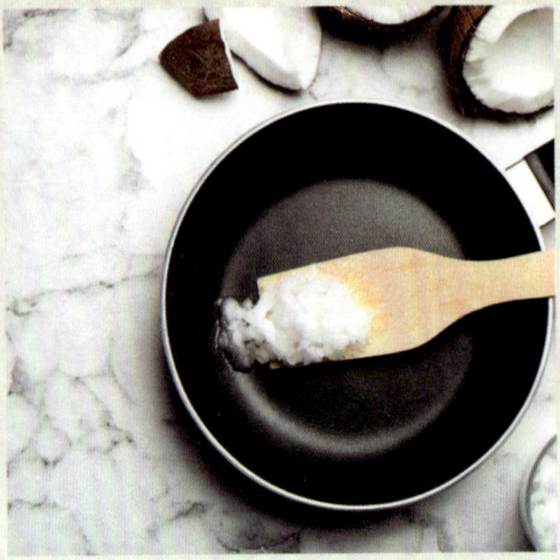

1 Always refer back to your first bath bomb and make sure you've got your work surface ready and all your equipment to hand.

2 Boil the kettle. Once boiled add 1 tablespoon of ground coffee to a microwavable mug and pour in a tiny splash of boiling water. Just enough to melt the coffee and create a thick paste.

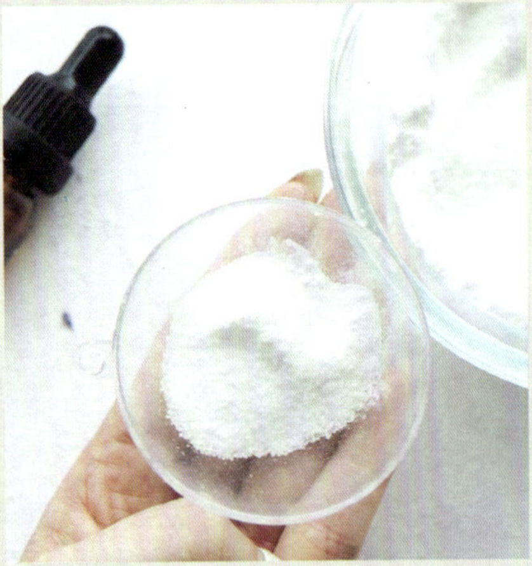

3 Add 1 tablespoon of coconut oil to your coffee paste and microwave for 60 seconds or until the mixture is completely liquified. Make sure to only microwave 20 seconds at a time so you can check on progress.

4 In your mixing bowl, add the bicarbonate of soda, cream of tartar, corn starch and Epsom salt before mixing thoroughly.

5 Pour your coffee oil mixture into your dry mix and stir quickly.

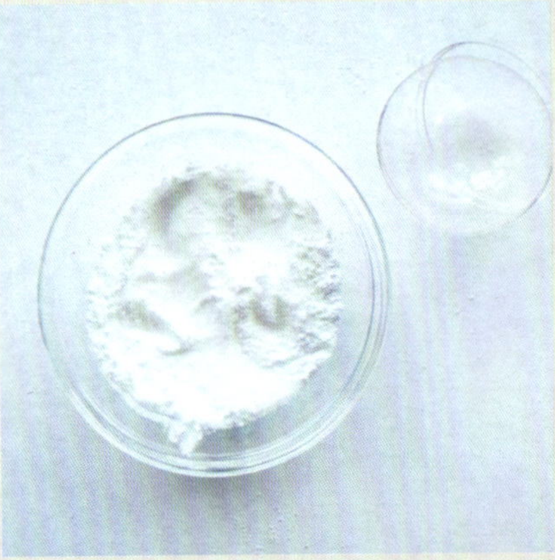

6 Once the two mixtures are combined, give it a mix with your hands to ensure it's all mixed together (you don't want any lumps). Don't forget you can always add more bicarb or water until you get that wet sand consistency.

7 Take a few coffee beans and place them in the centre of one of your bath bomb moulds with the smooth side facing up.

9 Start to compact your bath bomb moulds and fill again just above the rim - the same as you did in your first project.

10 Place your moulds together and hold for 10 - 15 seconds. Wrap in clingfilm and leave overnight.

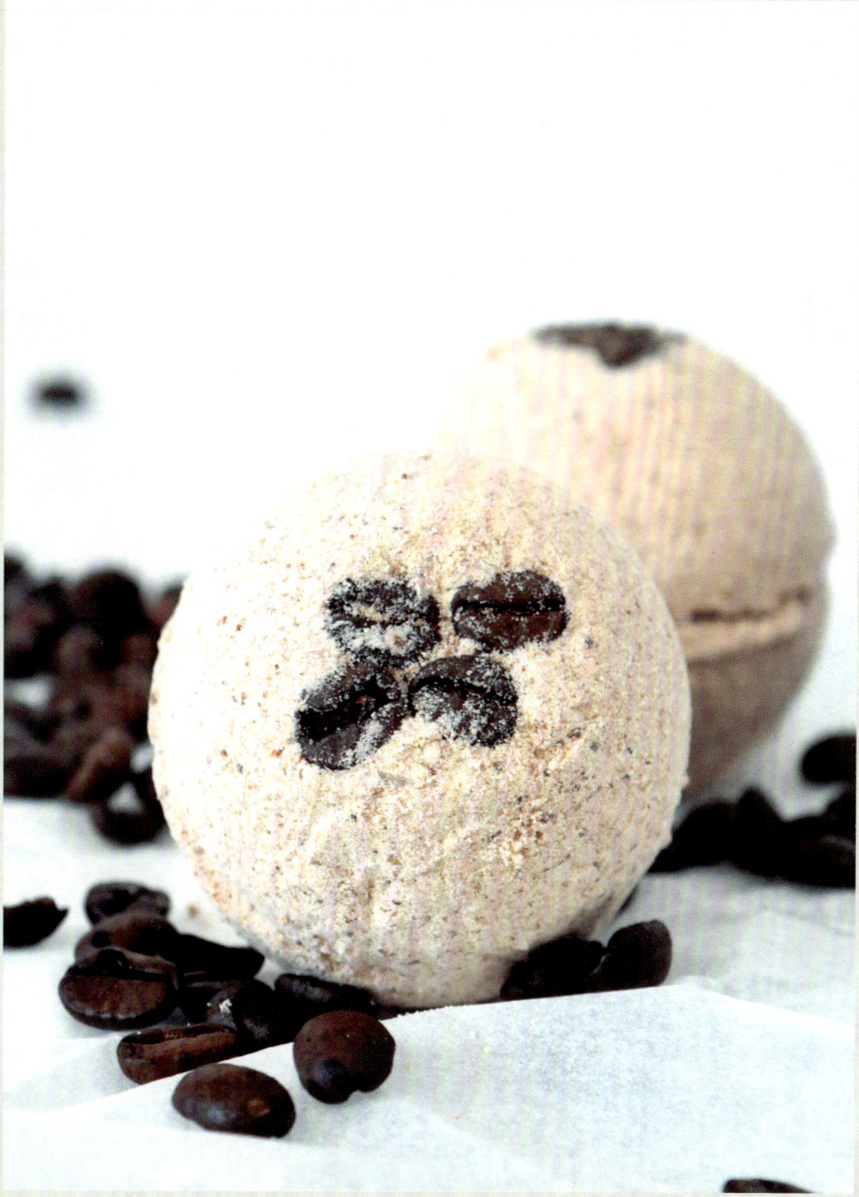

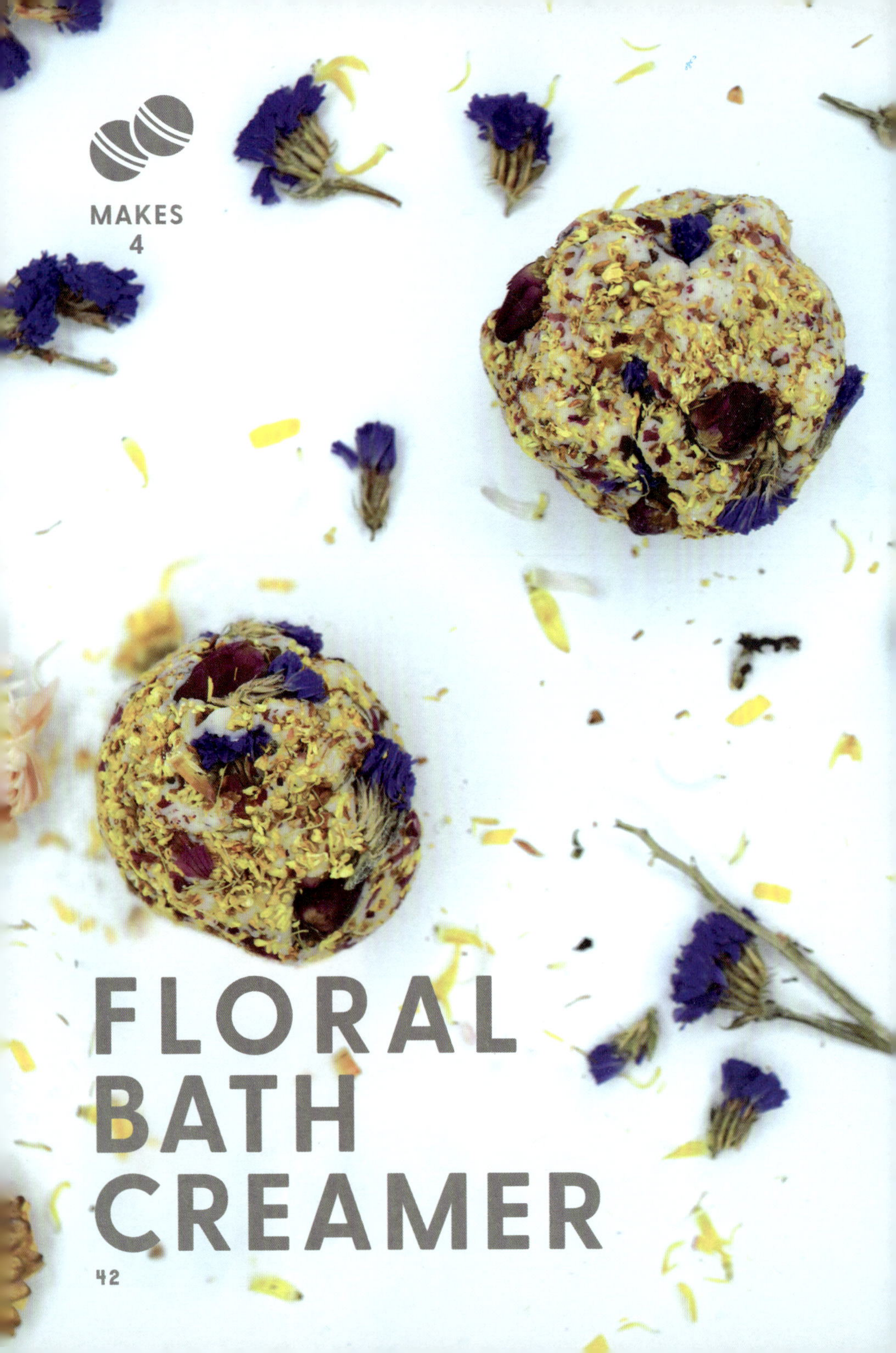

MAKES
4

FLORAL BATH CREAMER

FLORAL BATH CREAMER

The ideal mix between a bath melt and fizzy bath bomb. Whether you use cocoa or shea butter, these bath creamers will leave your skin feeling hydrated and nourished after your bath.

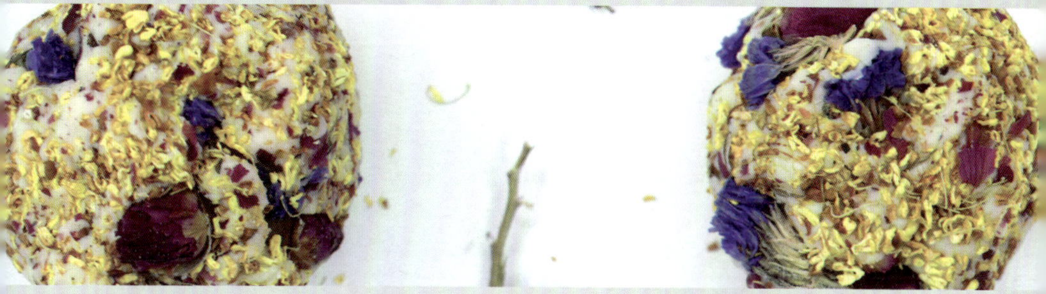

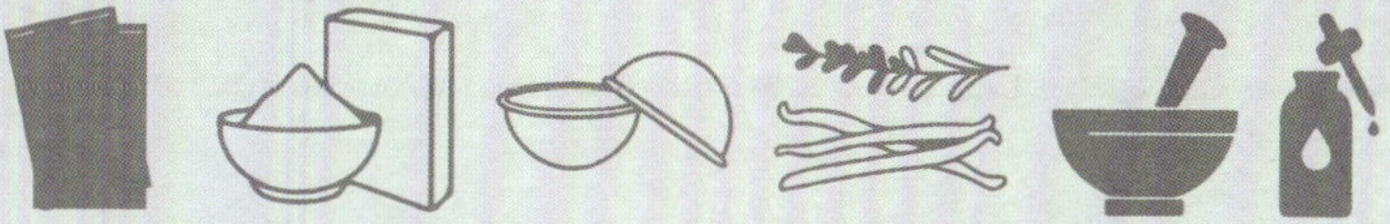

YOU WILL NEED

- A mixing bowl
- Microwave
- Microwavable Jug
- Whisk
- 2 x Bath Bomb moulds
- Clingfilm

INGREDIENTS

- Bicarbonate of Soda 100g
- Cocoa/Shea butter 70g
- Cream of Tartar 30g
- Corn Starch 50g
- Milk Powder 50g
- Coconut Oil 2 tablespoons
- 8–10 drops of essential oil
- Dried Flowers of your choice

METHOD

1 Always refer back to your first bath bomb and make sure you've got your work surface ready and all your equipment to hand.

2 For this recipe, you want to heat the mixture slowly to avoid the butters from burning. Fill a saucepan with 1-2 inches of water.

3 In your heatproof mixing bowl, add your cocoa or shea butter and coconut oil and place it on top of the pan of water.

4 Turn the heat on low to bring the water to a simmer and to melt your oil mixture. Don't forget to keep stirring until the mix has fully melted.

5 Safely remove your hot oil mix from the heat and pour into a heat proof jug.

6 Stir in your chosen essential oils and let it cool for a couple of minutes.

7 In your mixing bowl, add the bicarbonate of soda, cream of tartar, corn starch and milk powder and whisk them together until fully mixed.

8 Slowly add your butter oil mix to the dry ingredients, whisking as you pour.

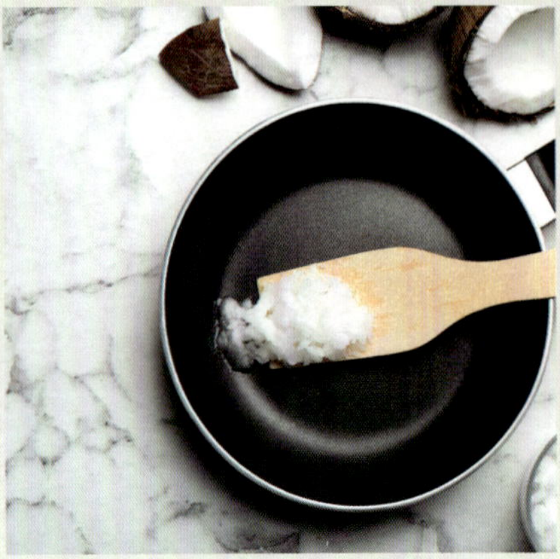

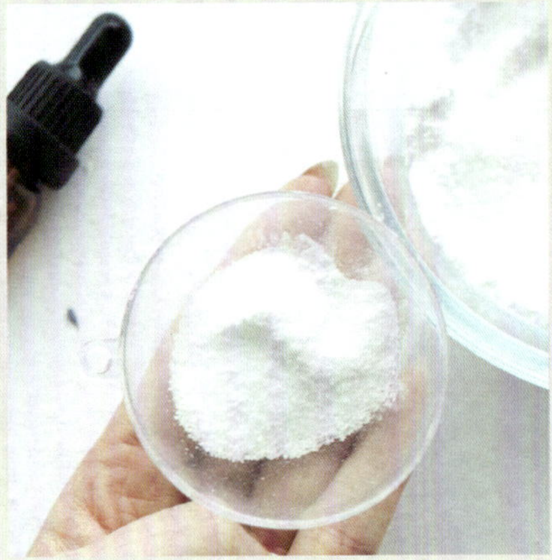

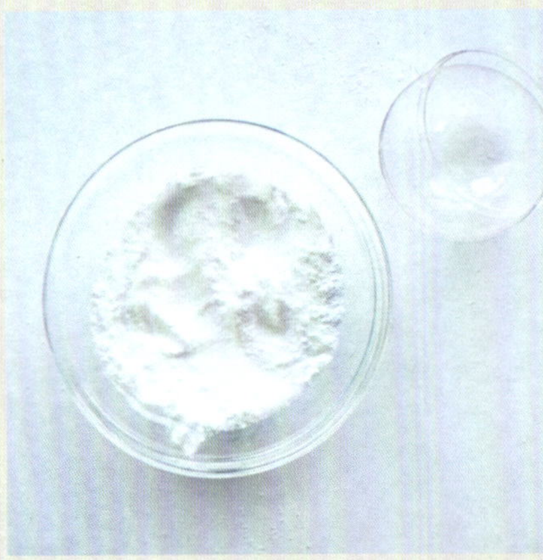

9 Once added, use your hands to mix into a dough that's easy to shape. When it's done it should feel oily and slightly sticky to touch.

10 Lay your dried flowers on a sheet of baking paper, making sure you have an even layer of flowers.

11 Grab a handful of the mixture and roll it into a ball shape. If the mix is too wet, add a small handful of bicarbonate of soda, if it is too dry melt a small spoon of coconut oil and add to the mix.

12 Roll your ball in the dried flowers, they should stick to it creating an outer coating of flowers.

13 Place your bath creamer in 1 half of a bath bomb mould before placing in the fridge for 1 hour. After you have removed from the fridge, keep them in the moulds and store in a well ventilated room for a further 24 hours.

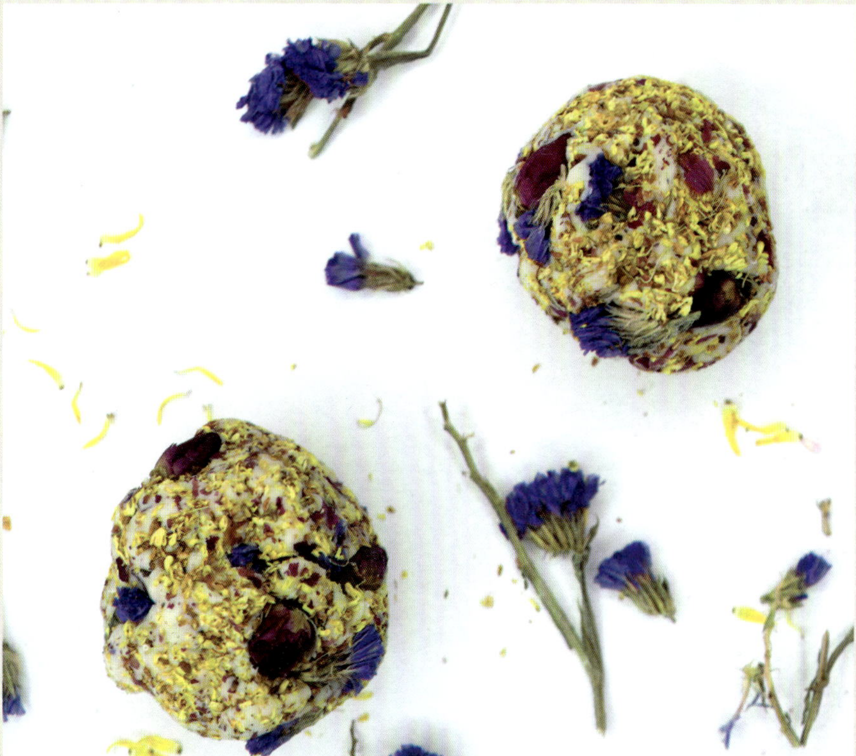

MAKES
4 - 6

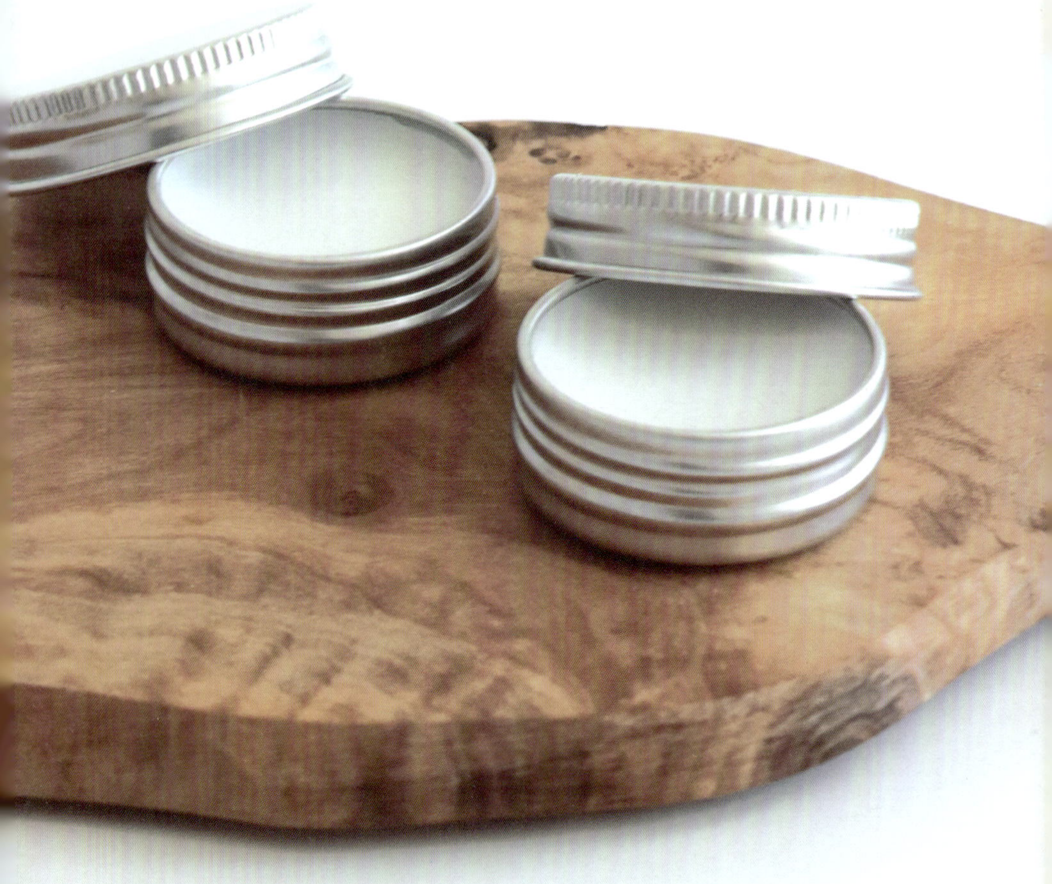

LIP BALM

LIP BALM

Help keep your lips hydrated with your very own lip balms. Bees wax has a number of health benefits from helping to treat eczema to acne prone skin. It also leaves your lips hydrated due to it's added moisture benefits!

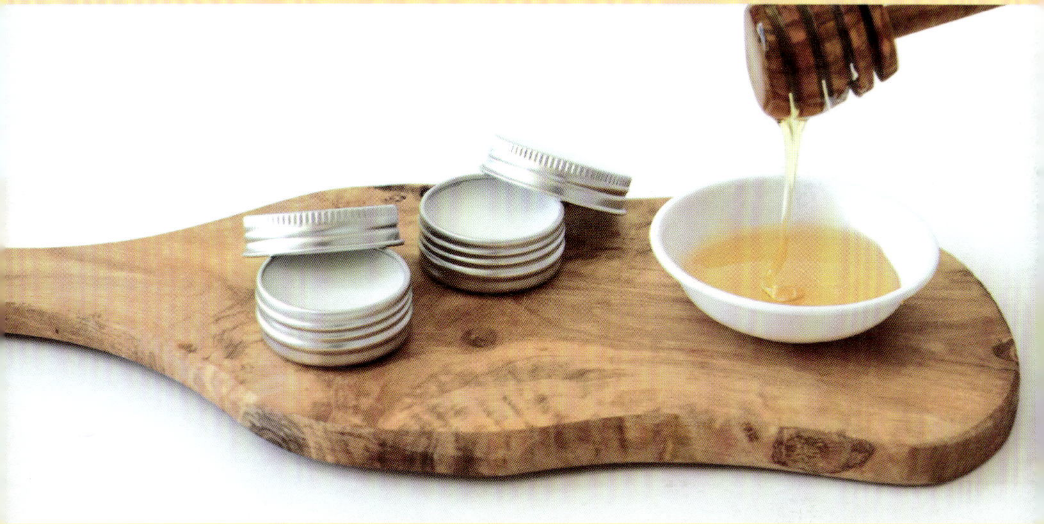

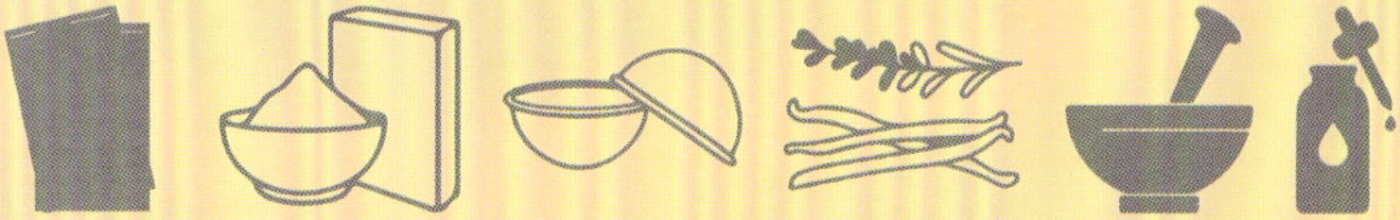

YOU WILL NEED

- 6 Metal tin/lip balm containers
- Microwavable jug
- Spoon/Stirrer

INGREDIENTS

- Beeswax: 1 – 2 tablespoons
- Essential Oil: 2 drops
- Coconut Oil: 1 – 2 tablespoons

METHOD

1 Prepare your work surface and equipment in the same way you did on the bath bomb projects.

2 Add equal parts beeswax and coconut oil to a microwavable jug and microwave for 2 minutes or until fully melted.

3 Once fully melted, add your chosen essential oil and stir. Be careful not to add too much as you don't want this to be overpowering.

4 Carefully pour the liquid mixture into your chosen container.

5 Let them set for 30 minutes before placing a lid on them.

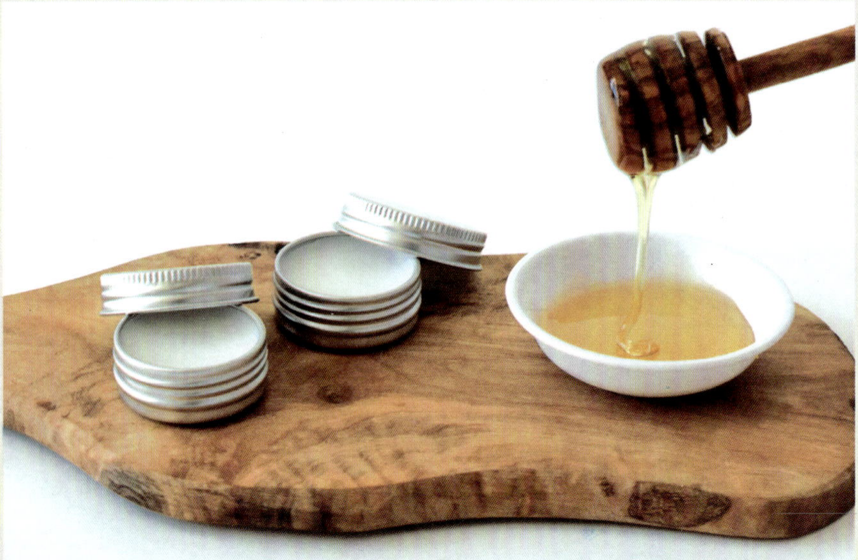